RUNNING A PRACTICE

D1807567

A MANUAL OF PRACTICE MANAGEMENT

SECOND EDITION

R.V.H. JONES, K.J. BOLDEN,
D.J. PEREIRA GRAY and M.S. HALL

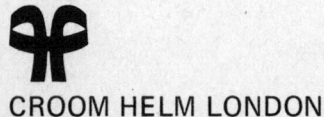

CROOM HELM LONDON

©1978 R.V.H. Jones, K.J. Bolden, D.J. Pereira Gray and M.S. Hall
Second Edition © 1981 R.V.H. Jones, K.J. Bolden, D.J. Pereira Gray and M.S. Hall
Croom Helm Ltd, 2-10 St John's Road, London SW11

British Library Cataloguing in Publication Data

Running a practice. – 2nd ed.
1. Medical offices – Management
2. Medical offices – Great Britain – Management
3. Family medicine – Great Britain
I. Jones, R V H
658'.91'36210425   R728

ISBN 0-7099-1410-6

Printed in Great Britain by
Biddles Ltd, Guildford, Surrey

CONTENTS

Contents

Part Seven: Organisation

Appendices

ACKNOWLEDGEMENTS

We should like to express our gratitude to the following for their help and advice: Professor G. Duncan Mitchell, Professor of Sociology, University of Exeter; Dr Trevor Hoskins, Hon. Sec. of the Medical Officers of Schools Association; Dr D. Buchanan, Assistant Scottish Secretary of the British Medical Association; N.O.J. Holberton, Devon Family Practitioner Committee and D. Mullins, chartered accountant.

We should also like to record our appreciation of the advice and helpful criticism given by Drs J.A.S. Forman, S. Jane Richards and Peter Selley.

We are grateful to the Editor of the *Journal of the Royal College of General Practitioners* for permission to publish those parts of the chapter on the Independent Contractor which have already appeared in his journal.

Finally our secretaries, especially Mrs Avis Hilder, who have survived indecipherable tapes and indescribable writing, deserve our grateful thanks.

PREFACE

As part of the Vocational Training Scheme at Exeter trainees are offered a practice management course during their final year. Originally planned as a practical course it was soon found necessary to explain the philosophy which underlies the working arrangements and decision-making in our own practices. The lack of reference material for such a course has prompted the production of this book. As we take joint responsibility for the views expressed, chapters have not been attributed to individuals.

We hope that trainees, trainers, and possibly others, may find something of interest.

PREFACE TO THE SECOND EDITION

The preparation of a second edition has enabled us to correct some errors, to revise and expand the chapters on records and audit, and to introduce new chapters on practice accounts and the training practice.

We hope that the usefulness of the book as an introduction to practice management will have been enhanced.

R.V.H.J.
K.J.B.
D.J.P.G.
M.S.H.

INTRODUCTION

The title phrase 'running a practice' was chosen to indicate that the contents of this book would be an overall view of all those activities which are involved in the day-to-day and longer-term organisation of a practice within the National Health Service. This is a large and complex subject. We have deliberately chosen to concentrate on principles rather than detail so that consideration can be given to all major topics within a relatively small volume. Descriptions of forms and office procedures have been given by Drury and Helen Owen. Further specific subjects are frequently covered in articles and supplements in the medical press.

For a general practitioner the ability to run his practice efficiently has certain direct and obvious advantages. He knows where he is—the surgeries are not overbooked, all forms and equipment are to hand, he can plan his half-days and holidays, the accounts are straightforward and up to date. His income is higher, with claim forms for items of service being filled in correctly and submitted without delay, mileage allowances are noted, bills are paid and reimbursements claimed at times which increase cash flow. The atmosphere in which he works is pleasant and friendly.

There are, however, other advantages for patients and doctors which are not so immediately apparent. Practice management and organisation are usually considered as distinct from clinical care. When lectures are given or courses are held for general practitioners the subject matter is either clinical or practice management. Rarely is any connection made between the two. Yet there is a direct relationship. Poor management inevitably results in a lower standard of clinical care. If staff are unhappy with their contracts (or lack of them), if partners are unhappy about their working conditions and do not meet to agree how things might be improved, if requests for visits are mislaid, messages lost, forms not available or wrongly filled in, the frustration and unhappiness in the practice spills over into relationships with patients. If through lack of organisation doctors are rushed or their surgeries are impossibly full, they become resentful and the care their patients receive is bound to suffer. If records are a shambles patients may be in danger of being given a drug to which they are sensitive, or a child fail to receive a booster because his immunisation state is unrecorded.

There is no doubt in our minds that in order to deliver a high standard of clinical care, clinical work must be backed up by good practice organisation.

There is also no doubt that one of the skills of practice management is to make sure that in spite of its complexity the practice runs smoothly, that the hum of activity arising from the organisation should be inaudible to the patient. If, as we believe, general practice should provide each patient with continuing personal care, it should be in a friendly calm atmosphere in which as far as possible the patient feels at ease and at home. Hustle bustle and over-busyness diminish patients. One aim of a patient-orientated practice should be to keep its necessarily complex organisation out of sight. In the following pages we describe the various behind-the-scenes activities which are involved in running a practice within the National Health Service.

References

Drury, M. *The Medical Secretary's Handbook*, 3rd edition (London: Baillière Tindall, 1975).
Owen, H. *Administration in General Practice* (London: E. Arnold, 1975).

PART ONE: THE SCENE

1 THE NATURE OF GENERAL PRACTICE

There are two main kinds of doctor: those who are primarily interested in diseases and those who are primarily interested in people. Perhaps the most important decision of all for any young doctor, before, during and after qualification, is to identify his own characteristics and to become quite certain in which category he or she is. Both types of doctor are essential for the future of medical practice. Both undertake equally valuable work.

For the disease-centred doctor the kind of disease the patient has is the central focus of his interest and care, and the particular person who happens to have it is inevitably the secondary consideration. By contrast for patient-centred doctors the patient, his personality, his attitudes, his family and home are of central interest and the particular kind of disease he happens to have at the time is important but secondary.

The crucial importance of this distinction is that doctors in one category usually do not feel completely at home if they are practising the other branch of medicine.

Most trainees if they are undertaking a three-year programme of training for general practice will have already decided that they are patient-centred doctors. Many will have doubts, however, and some will have serious misgivings. It is important that these are voiced and discussed.

Variety in General Practice

People sometimes talk about general practice as if it is a uniform whole, which can be discussed and debated as if it has fixed and common characteristics. The opposite is of course the case and one of the main characteristics of general practice is its extreme diversity. No two practices are quite the same and even in the same road adjacent practices may have totally different attitudes and standards.

All those entering general practice must begin to understand some of the reasons for the variety. These conveniently come under the headings of: people, place, premises, partner(s) and personality.

1. People

Medicine is a service. The purpose of medical care is to bring to the

17

people in any society a medical service appropriate to their needs.
It follows that the first essential in considering any health system is to
test the appropriateness of the service in relation to the needs of the
people as perceived by themselves and by the health professionals. This
principle holds true in general practice and one of the main causes of
variety in general practice is the variety of people themselves.
Obvious examples are race, social class, and age structure.

Race. Culture has an immense influence on attitudes towards illness
and on attitudes to the process of seeking help. The presence of significant numbers of people of a different race as patients will have a
major impact on the pattern of a general practice. Changes in the
racial pattern of the locality will alter the character of the practices in
that locality.

Social Class. The tremendous significance of social class in relation to
illness is little appreciated from hospitals, but there is overwhelming
evidence that social class is one of the main determinants of morbidity,
mortality, and the use of health services. Life expectation at every age
is significantly less in the lower social classes from the perinatal period
to old age. People in social class five on average die younger than those
in social class one. In analysing the people who are the patients in a
practice, the numbers and properties and the different social classes
greatly influence the nature of the work in that practice (DHSS, 1976).

Age. Similarly, the age of a patient is another major determinant of
illness (Fry, 1977). Not only do elderly people often develop several
disabilities simultaneously but their increasing loss of independence,
frailty and loss of mobility mean that they have a disproportionately
high home visiting rate. In some practices on the south coast of England
the proportion of all patients who are over the age of 65 is more than
one third whereas in other towns it may be as low as 5 per cent. The
distribution of age of the patients of the practice therefore is another
cause of variety in general practice.

2. The Place

General practice has long been close to the people and indeed is a
community service in a community setting. All general practices to some
extent absorb the pattern of living of people in that area and hence there
are wide variations between practices in, say, a Welsh mining village,
the centre of Liverpool, and a practice on Dartmoor. Because the

problems of people's lives impinge on us and indeed may dominate, the problems of people living in different places will be reflected in the general practitioner's consulting-room. The place where the practice *is* will inevitably determine to a large extent the pattern of practice.

3. Provision

Although general practice may be the most isolated and individual medical branch of the health service, general practitioners do not practise alone. The quality of the work that they can do, whether in single-handed practice or a big partnership, must always depend to a considerable extent on the provision of other health services in the neighbourhood. Whether or not there is a general-practitioner hospital, whether or not there is a general-practitioner maternity unit, whether or not the local social services department is coping well with its work-load, whether or not the provision of health visitors and nurses is adequate, will govern the use by practitioners of these services and hence their pattern of practice. In understanding how, and why, a practice works and what its potential is for further improvement, the provision of other health and social services in the neighbourhood must therefore be taken into consideration.

4. Premises

The premises used for general medical practice changed little in the nineteenth century, but a dramatic revolution occurred in the middle of the twentieth century. One of the most obvious signs of this radical review of primary care was the transformation of general-practitioner premises. It can now be seen that getting the premises correct was rightly one of the first targets for the reorganisation of general practice that took place in the 1960s (BMA Charter, 1965).

Whatever the skills, hopes, attitudes, or aspirations of the doctor he needs a place to exercise his skills. For example, if there is no treatment-room it is difficult to realise the full potential of both attached nurses and practice nurses. The simple criterion of whether or not there is a treatment-room is one of the great indicators of the range of activities which can take place in practices. Many practices without treatment-rooms will refer to hospital conditions which doctors and nurses working together can often manage, and manage excellently, in a properly equipped nursing sister's room.

The presence of a common-room can similarly subtly alter the relationships between partners and other members of general-practice teams. The Scottish Council for Postgraduate Medical Education (1977)

lists the presence of a common-room as one of the factors now expected
in training practices. They believe that the presence of a library in the
common-room and the ability of partners to meet on neutral ground is
of special value in promoting partnership discussion and relationships.
It is not, of course, true that without a common-room partners cannot
meet and discuss; in many such practices close partnership relationships
exist. Nevertheless, in our experience having a room where partners can
meet independently of another partner being held up and running late,
or having to fit in an extra patient or medical, is a great boon; it
promotes relaxed discussion over coffee and may be a convenient setting
for regular meetings of partners and, say, a weekly lunch. Such meetings
are particularly important in bigger partnerships.

It is difficult to assess how irritating it can be if partners do not have
their own consulting-rooms, which is still the case in many general
practices today. Practices which have been able to provide each partner
with a separate room make it possible for consulting-rooms to be
furnished much more personally, and for them to reflect the personality
of the doctor.

Finally, there is no doubt that many of the future developments in
general practice will depend upon improved methods of record-keeping
and the introduction of new systems of organisation of records including,
for example, such basic methods as age/sex registers and diagnostic
indexes. All these systems take up room and it is becoming clear that
those practices which have enough room to organise efficient systems
of handling information are becoming able to offer a better standard of
care for their patients. It follows that the presence of an adequate size
secretarial office, or better still a second office, may be a condition for
improving the standard of clinical care.

5. Partners

We analyse in the Conclusion the significance of the partnership relationship to general practitioners. Of all the factors involved in choosing a
new practice, we advise trainees to place the greatest weight on being
sure of compatibility of personality with partners. The partnership
relationship is a form of professional marriage, and there is no doubt
that the ability to practise a high standard of clinical care depends on
the quality of care, the attitude and the standard of one's partners. Even
in those practices in which separate lists are maintained, and in which
patients identify with a particular partner, it is always true that there
will be some cross-over between partners and patients and inevitably
partners will see one's patients in the evenings, during holidays and study

leave. Furthermore, partners will be responsible for forming the
philosophy of the practice which will influence and outwardly govern
the attitudes and behaviour of the practice secretaries, receptionists, and
the health visitor and nurses. The feeling of the group of partners which
is so difficult to express is the average picture that the partners convey
to their working colleagues.

No matter what the ideals and skills of a new incoming partner, the
ultimate effect he will have on his patients will be determined to an
extent greater than he perhaps realises by the other partners in the
practice. Furthermore, in a close working relationship over the years,
partners increasingly influence each other. There is no reasonable hope
of expecting to change two or three senior partners in their views. They
are much more likely to change the views of the lonely isolated incoming
partner. The tradition and history of a practice has a strong influence on
its organisation and philosophy. The presence of different practice
traditions is a further factor underlying the variety found in general
practice.

6. *The Doctor's Personality*

One of the landmarks of modern general practice was the publication of
Balint's book, *The Doctor, His Patient and the Illness* in 1957. It has
been said (*Journal of the Royal College of General Practitioners*, 1972)
'Balint will become for general practice what Freud has become for
psychiatry', that is to say he will be seen as a great prophet who introduced a major new dimension to a discipline. Whilst it is absurd to
suggest the psychoanalytical approach of Freud is the 'be all and end
all' of psychiatry, it is impossible to deny that the whole development
of modern psychiatry has been influenced by his views.

Similarly, it is quite possible to agree that much of modern general
practice does not depend upon Balint, but it is equally impossible to
deny that his views have influenced, and decisively influenced, the last
twenty-five years of development of the discipline of general practice.

One of the key ideas which Balint introduced was that much of the
care provided in general practice depended on the personality of the
doctor himself. He expressed this in the model by saying that the
doctor was the most important 'drug' used in general practice; and
followed it through by saying that doctors who wished to practise
family medicine must learn to understand their own personalities, to
understand the side-effects of the use of this drug, and the indications
for appropriate use. Even twenty-five years later this message has not
yet been generally understood, and many general practitioners still

enter general practice, either untrained or having attended courses of vocational training, without learning this essential fact. In order to be good general practitioners we must first understand ourselves. We must understand the strength and weakness of our own personalities, the way we affect other people, and the way we cope with some of our more important inner feelings.

There are many ways of obtaining these insights, but the simplest and most effective appears to be by a series of discussions with one's peers, preferably led by someone who is experienced in the analysis of personality and inter-personal behaviour. The traditional psychoanalytical school believed that general practitioners obtained these insights best if led by a professionally trained psychoanalyst, such as Balint himself, and this school has continued until the present time. Others have increasingly wondered if general practitioners could not themselves lead groups and assist their colleagues in obtaining similar insights.

Many vocational training schemes including those at Ipswich and at Exeter are now firmly based on the concept of continuing small group discussion as an essential method of helping trainees understand their own personality. By working with a group of colleagues, by arguing and struggling with knowledge, ideas and attitudes, trainees over a long period of time (preferably three years) begin to understand the importance of human behaviour, learn to tolerate their colleagues' idiosyncrasies, and more important still begin to understand how their colleagues tolerate them.

These insights we believe are essential if a general practitioner is to be able to cope with the tremendous variety of behaviour which will be presented to him by patients who are, or think they may be, ill. Without such training, anger in the doctor is common, and it is striking how angry trainees or young principals may become when patients behave in ways which they have hitherto assumed were inappropriate. Only by facing such behaviour among one's peers can one learn to recognise patterns which make the doctor angry, and begin to understand a patient's feelings. Among the educational aims of the Exeter course learning to feel what it is like to be a patient is one of the highest on the list.

Recordon (1972) has said that doctors eventually get the patients that they deserve, and it is probably true that over a period of at least a dozen years or more there will be a progressive trend for patients of certain types and categories to collect on any particular doctor's list. In order to understand this phenomenon it is necessary to understand the personality of the general practitioner. If, for example, he has a particular interest in a particular disease, whether organic or psychological, he is likely to detect it earlier and to treat it more effectively if only because he is more interested and gives more of himself. He tends to collect patients with such a condition by recommendation and referral. If on the other hand, he is uncomfortable with patients who express anger or fear, he will over the years gradually lose such patients, or lose contact with them as they seek the outlets they need from other doctors or other sources. Thus over a period of time the doctor will see more and more of what he is interested in, and less and less of what he is least efficient at detecting or managing.

Whilst this may lead to contentment over the years, it can also lead to a fall in standards if the doctor is not confronted periodically with evidence of those aspects of care in which he still has most to learn. Developing a tolerant partnership relationship is one of the ways in which the small group of the partners meeting together may be able to assist each other in such aspects of medicine.

Most doctors have inner needs to dominate people, and may succeed in establishing dominant relationships with large numbers of their patients. Others have a need to be loved, and will over the years collect large numbers of patients who will fulfil this emotional need. Ultimately each general practitioner must ask himself the question whether or not he needs to be respected, or needs to be loved; most of us fall into one or other of these categories. This can be a helpful analysis in aiding a young doctor to determine in which aspects of care he or she is likely to be relatively strong or weak.

The personality of the doctor is thus of special importance. It is the key to successful personal medical care. The variety found among general practitioners' personalities is one of the main causes of the variety found in general practice.

References and Further Reading

Balint, M. *The Doctor, His Patient and the Illness*, 2nd edition (London: Pitman, 1964).
British Medical Association Charter (London: BMA, 1965).
Department of Health and Social Security. *Prevention and Health: Everybody's Business* (London: HMSO, 1976).
Fry, J. James Mackenzie Lecture 1976. *Journal of the Royal College of General Practitioners*, 26 (1977), pp. 9-17.
Journal of the Royal College of General Practitioners. Editorial, Michael Balint. 22 (1972), pp. 133-5.

Recordon, P. *Journal of the Royal College of General Practitioners*, 22 (1972), pp. 818-27.
Scottish Council for Postgraduate Medical Education. *Training in General Practice* (Edinburgh: SCPME, 1977).

2 THE GENERAL PRACTITIONER AS AN INDEPENDENT CONTRACTOR

The variety found within general practice is the result of many different factors. This diversity is in turn shown in many different ways—in the number and type of staff employed, in the scale and type of premises used, in the standards of furnishing and equipment, and in the way in which the practice is organised.

This is only possible because general practitioners are free under their contracts with the Family Practitioner Committee (or Health Board in Scotland or N. Ireland) to provide services for their patients in the way that they consider most appropriate, subject to certain safeguards.

They are, in fact, independent contractors. If they were not so but were instead employees of the Area or Regional Health Authority (as are hospital specialists and community physicians) then this book would be superfluous—because in that case responsibility for staff, premises, equipment and services provided would be the responsibility of the employing authorities (AHA and RHA) and not of the individual general practitioner.

This term 'independent contractor' has given rise to enormous confusion and misunderstanding. Many hospital specialists do not understand its implications. Many patients think general practitioners are civil servants employed by the government, and many general practitioners themselves are dubious about their own independence. The term applies to any self-employed individual, whether he is in business or a profession, who agrees to provide a service for another individual. He agrees (contracts) to provide the service himself or through his employees. He does this on his own responsibility and is not employed by some other person or organisation to do it. In other words, he is independent.

Self-employed plumbers, lawyers, dentists, chemists, opticians, are all independent contractors. They are free to run their business or arrange their professional practice as they wish. They may practise singly or in partnership. They may belong to associations of likeminded businessmen or professionals. They may subscribe to codes of practice laid down by their fellows. But for each independent contractor the two sides of the same coin are:

(a) *freedom* to organise his own business as he deems appropriate (this results in variety and flexibility);

(b) *responsibility* for the adequateness of the service he provides for his patient/client/customer.*

In the chapters which follow the main components of practice organisation for which general practitioners are responsible owing to their independent contractor status are discussed.

The Contract

In some professions or trades there is no written contract between the customer and the provider of the service. In others there are either specific contracts or conditions under which a contract is held to have been undertaken in law. When negotiating with builders, for example, an accepted estimate is a recognised form of contract. The contract between a general practitioner and an individual patient begins when a general practitioner accepts that patient on his list. The services which he is expected to provide for that patient depend on whether the general practitioner has contracted with the Family Practitioner Committee (or Health Board) for the provision of general medical services, for maternity services, or for contraceptive services.

When a general practitioner signs his contract with the Family Practitioner Committee, the FPC is, on behalf of the government, fulfilling its basic medical function of ensuring that each individual who lives within its area has access to adequate primary medical care. In order to do this, it has to know from where the general practitioner intends to practise, that the premises are satisfactory, that he will be available for consultation at defined times, and that his off-duty arrangements will not leave his patients inadequately cared for. These constraints within which a general practitioner practises in the NHS do inevitably limit his freedom in that he is not free to practise from totally inadequate premises in such a way that his patients receive totally inadequate care. But these constraints do not make him any less independent than the industrialist whose factory must pass certain health regulations, or the owner of a guest-house whose building has to satisfy fire regulations.

*In all organisations (commercial, professional or NHS) the total service provided is dependent on the financial resources, i.e. on the money available. The responsibility of the independent contractor operates within the available financial limits. (Ed.)

Practical Consequences

1. One main consequence of the fact that general practitioners are independent contractors is that both patients and doctor have a choice. Not only can the patient choose which general practitioner to go to but by mutual agreement the contract can be a continuing one over many years. This chance of generally maintaining or continuing a relationship is not possible in those countries where the doctor whom a patient sees for his primary medical care is a salaried employee and has no contracts with individual patients.

The fact that the general practitioner has a personal and usually continuing relationship with his individual patients makes his responsibility for the organisation of his practice and the standard of care which he provides a personal one also.

2. Secondly, in addition to his clinical responsibilities the general practitioner has administrative and financial responsibilities within his practice. The complexities of administration and finance are continually increasing. The training of most general practitioners has until recently failed to recognise that a general practitioner has managerial responsibilities. The consequence of this attitude has been that most general practitioners have a long way to go before their practices can be objectively judged as efficient by current business standards.

3. Thirdly, as self-employed independent contractors, general practitioners are taxed under Schedule D rather than Schedule E. The significance of this is discussed in Chapter 9.

4. Fourthly, as independent contractors our ability to influence the conditions under which we work and the services which our patients receive is immeasurably greater than would pertain if we were employees. It is up to us whether we work in pleasant rooms or drab, in warm rooms or cold, with efficient help or none, whether we have a larger or smaller car, a calculator or an abacus. With regard to services the independent contractor is free to choose the range of clinical activities that he offers above the basic contract; whether, for example, he does minor surgery, ECGs, manipulation or holds well-baby clinics.

The practical consequence of these freedoms is that each general practitioner must be aware of the results that his actions may have on practice organisation and finance, as well as practice standards. It is essential that there should be agreement between partners concerning priorities and policies.

Contrast between Independent Contractors and Salaried Employees

The characteristics of independent contractors and the services they give, namely those of personal responsibility, variety and flexibility, have been contrasted with the services provided by salaried employees.

Recently Gray (1977) has discussed in more detail the relationships between the ways in which people work and the effect this has on the ways in which the needs of clients are met. He pointed out that in a large firm or government office employees are usually arranged in a hierarchy — with responsibility to the person above them in the hierarchy and ultimately to their employer rather than to the client. In such hierarchies anonymity is encouraged (e.g. 'all correspondence should be addressed to the head of department') and responsibility is corporate rather than personal. Continuity of service in a hierarchy is haphazard and depends on chance — the customer/client sees whoever happens to be behind the desk or wielding the patellar hammer on that particular afternoon. The authoritarian nature of a hierarchy encourages employees to behave in an authoritarian way to clients. Such large organisations can only function efficiently if there is standardisation of policy and rigid rules of procedure.

All these characteristics are in direct contrast to the requirements of patients in general practice. Surveys (Hill *et al.*, 1968, Gray, 1979, Lawson, 1980) have confirmed that these requirements include as top priority the presence of an accessible family doctor whom they have chosen, who has personal responsibility for their medical care and who gets to know them and their family over a period of time. Increasingly the relationship between patient and general practitioner is one of negotiation rather than authority. In Appendix A a more detailed comparison of the differences between independent contractors and salaried employees is presented in tabular form.

The more detailed the analysis of the role of a general practitioner, the more closely does the work expected of him (Leeuwenhorst Working Party definition) correspond to that provided by independent contractors rather than the pattern of work and behaviour imposed on salaried employees by the character of the hierarchy in which they work.

As partnerships grow larger and single-handed practices become less common, it is an interesting point to consider at what size a practice with its ancillary staff is in danger of assuming the characteristics of a hierarchy so that the face presented to the patient becomes indistinguishable from that presented in the Post Office or Gas showrooms. In one large practice Forman (1971), conscious of this danger, has described how in a practice with eight partners the practice was subdivided into a number of self-contained working units each comprising two doctors, supporting staff, and a list of their own patients.

Tailpiece

In view of the foregoing discussion and the continuing debate both inside and outside the profession on the merits or otherwise of general practitioners being independent contractors, it is interesting to note (Jones, 1978) that primary medical care is provided by independent contractors in all countries of the EEC despite many differences in methods of payment and contracts of service. In each country individual patients contract with individual doctors for their primary medical care.

We believe that it is in the best interests of both patients and doctors that this position should continue. Both the BMA (1976) and the RCGP (1977) strongly supported the continuance of the independent-contractor status in their evidence to the Royal Commission. However, it is under attack from the TUC (1977), the Royal College of Midwives (1977) and the Health Visitors' Association (1977).

Young doctors should in our opinion be aware of the importance of the issues involved. A change in the independent-contractor status of general practitioners working in the NHS would not only affect the remuneration of doctors but would also involve a fundamental change in the nature and delivery of primary medical care. It would alter the foundation of family doctoring.

References and Further Reading

British Medical Association. *Evidence to the Royal Commission on the NHS* (London: BMA, 1976).
Forman, J.A.S. *Update Plus*, 1 (1971), pp. 265-70.
Gray, D.J. Pereira. 'General Practitioners and the Independent Contractor Status', *Journal of the Royal College of General Practitioners*, 27 (1977), pp. 750-6.
——— 'The Key to Personal Care', *Journal of the Royal College of General Practitioners*, 29 (1979), pp. 666-78.
Health Visitors' Association. Evidence to the Royal Commission on the NHS. *Health Visitor*, 50 (1977), p. 75.
Hill, M., McAuley, R.G., Spaulding, W.B. & Wilson, M. *Canadian Medical Association Journal*, 98 (1968), pp. 734-8.
Jones, R.V.H. *Update*, 16 (1978), pp. 1503-15.

Lawson, R.J. *Journal of the Royal College of General Practitioners*, 30 (1980), pp. 137-8.

Leeuwenhorst Working Party. Statement of 'the work of the General Practitioner'. *Journal of the Royal College of General Practitioners*, 27 (1977), p. 117.

Royal College of General Practitioners. Evidence to the Royal Commission on the NHS. *Journal of the Royal College of General Practitioners*, 27 (1977), pp. 197-206.

Royal College of Midwives. Evidence to the Royal Commission on the NHS. *Nursing Times* (10 March 1977).

Trades Union Council. Evidence to the Royal Commission on the NHS (1977). Quoted in *BMA News Review* (October 1977), p. 343.

PART TWO: BUILDINGS

3 PREMISES: GENERAL CONSIDERATIONS

The general practitioner's most important skill may be his use of the consultation, and his most used instrument the pen, but both require somewhere to be exercised. Just as the style of one's practice is very much an individual matter, so also the type of premises often reflects the individualism of the general practitioner. What follows can only be a short description of the range of practice premises generally in use today.

The improvements in the methods of remuneration of family doctors in the 1966 Charter led to the introduction of notional rents, reimbursement of rates, improvement grants and a cost rent scheme designed to help finance new purpose-built premises. The establishment of the General Practice Finance Corporation at the same time provided one source of capital from which general practitioners could borrow to improve or build premises. Widespread improvement in the standard of medical practice premises has resulted.

1. The Basic Practice Unit

There are few general practices nowadays where the accommodation consists only of a waiting-room and consulting-room. For most doctors the basic practice unit consists of a room for the doctor, a room for the patients, and one for the office staff.

This basic practice accommodation can be extended in various ways, which reflect both the increased complexity of running a modern practice and also the increased range of procedures and services which nowadays are carried out under one roof. Many doctors prefer an examination-room separate from their consulting-room, whilst others prefer twin consulting/examination-rooms with easy communication between them. Treatment-rooms in which doctors, nurses or chiropodists may work, rooms for health visitors and speech therapists, and a staff common-room are other frequent additions.

Furthermore a teaching practice, or one intending to become a teaching practice, must consider the extra accommodation a trainee practitioner needs. Especially important is a room from which he can consult, and a quiet room or reading-room in which he may study.

In a large partnership it may be decided to work as subgroups, in which separate teams of doctor, receptionist, nurse and health visitor look after their own practice of patients. In such cases each subgroup may have its own waiting/reception area. Such a system, when used in large group practices, is said greatly to improve continuity of care while at the same time relieving administration and communication (Forman, 1971).

2. Essential Requirements for Practice Premises

(a) Flow

An understanding of the movement of doctors, staff and patients around the premises is essential to good organisation. If a group of doctors is moving into new purpose-built premises, then it is advisable to study the movement in the old premises to try and get some idea of the needs of the new. Points to consider include — the frequency that corridors are used by more than one person at a time; whether particular areas are used by nurses carrying treatment trays, and if so, whether corridors are wide enough; whether the treatment-room is sufficiently central to be used to the maximum by the doctors.

It is nearly always impossible to meet all the ideal requirements for flow within the building. Often the waiting area becomes isolated from the consulting units and the treatment-room. If this is the case, then consideration should be given to the provision of small secondary waiting areas nearer to the consulting-rooms. For example, the doctor may consult with a patient and then decide that the patient needs to be seen in the treatment-room. In such cases, it is very useful to be able to tell the patient to go and wait in the subsidiary waiting area adjoining the treatment-room.

(b) Reception Area and Call System

The reception area is the hub of any medical centre and the design needs exceptionally careful thought to ensure a combination of efficiency, courtesy and privacy. A full discussion appears in Chapter 5.

If the flow of patients to and from doctors' consulting-rooms and the treatment areas is to work smoothly, the call system needs to be planned as an integral part of the overall practice strategy. A friendly reception service may be spoilt by a badly designed call system. Further discussion of this also appears in Chapter 5.

(c) Office and Telephone

The office, whilst of central importance to the whole practice, need
not occupy a central point in the building. Ease of access for doctors
and reception staff is of course desirable, but so too is the need to ensure
a quiet and relatively undisturbed area in which the medical secretaries
may work.

Telephone and internal communication systems are now so complex
and adaptable to individual requirements that expert advice from the
Post Office and commercial communication companies is advisable.
Chapter 5 discusses both these topics in more detail.

(d) Lavatories, Wash-rooms and Kitchens

The sign-posting and positioning of patients' toilets is most important.
It is a waste of staff time if they are constantly being interrupted to
direct patients to badly indicated lavatories. At least one toilet should
be of adequate size to admit a wheelchair and should adjoin the
treatment-room so that there can be a hatch-way through which
specimens can be passed directly to the treatment-room nurse. A special
'Specitest' lavatory/pan is available which takes a disposable urine
collection pot.

It should go without saying that adequate facilities for washing
should be available to patients and staff alike. Staff will appreciate a
larger room where they can have their own coat lockers. Facilities for
making tea and coffee are essential. Indeed larger premises may justify
a small kitchen where snack meals can be prepared for practice and
other meetings.

(e) Examination-rooms

Doctors differ in their attitude to their own consulting-room, in regard
to whether it should be a room for only talking with patients, or whether
examination of the patient should take place there as well. One of the
differences between hospital practice and general practice is in the realm
of consultation. Many practitioners feel that a non-clinical atmosphere
contributes to the success of the consultation. It follows from this that
some doctors may wish to separate the clinical examination of the
patient from the consultation.

If this is the case, then the facilities for clinical examination need to
be physically separate from but adjoining the consultation-room. If a
doctor wishes to see more than one patient at a time, then the problems
of sound-proofing make it essential for the consultation-room not to
have an inter-communicating door. Patients must be led into the

corridor and into a separate examination-room.

Various compromises on this theme are possible. It might be reasonable to have a consulting-room with an examination alcove, and with an adjoining examination-room so that the doctor could consult in a non-clinical atmosphere, and yet examine the patient in the clinical confines of the alcove whilst waiting for a further patient to undress in the examination-room proper adjoining the consulting-room.

3. Optional Requirements

An increased sophistication of services offered by general practitioners must lead to demands for specialised accommodation within the medical centre. Some of these 'optional extras' are dealt with below, and because primary care physicians are individuals and because different areas have different needs the list is not intended to be comprehensive.

(a) A Separate Treatment-room

A separate treatment-room is probably the commonest addition to the basic unit. Its size is determined both by the projected work-load of the practice and the staffing structure planned for the premises. Clearly a practice which employs practice nurses throughout the day will use the treatment-room far more than a practice without a nurse.

The room will need to have at least one examination couch. If there are several couches suitable screening can enable more than one patient to be seen at a time. This is specially useful where the nurse decides a patient should be seen by the doctor before a nursing procedure is completed. As sterilisation of instruments will be done in this room, in either a small autoclave or a steriliser, adequate ventilation is essential. A good adjustable light over one of the couches is important for minor surgical procedures and pelvic examination.

Suggestions for further reading which include consideration of design points for treatment-rooms are given at the end of this chapter.

(b) Pathological and Clinical Procedures

It is usual to carry out basic urinalysis and haematological investigations in the treatment-room, but such procedures can hinder the flow of patients and a small room designed for these purposes may be justified in larger practices.

Many practitioners find a haemoglobinometer, ESR tubes, and a peak flow meter useful for providing a quick answer when one is needed. Other more costly equipment includes an ECG machine, audiometer, a centrifuge, a microscope and an Ames photometer.

Unfortunately, British general practices have always been relatively poorly equipped. The reason is mainly because since 1948 there has never been, and still is not, any financial return on capital invested in equipment.

(c) Nurses' and Health Visitors' Rooms

All practices which believe in the value of the primary health care team should have an office which can be used by attached nurses and health visitors. The room need not be large, but should be equipped with a desk, cupboards and filing space. Its use should be agreed before occupancy. For example, is it for private use by the nurses and health visitors or may patients be seen there as well? Who can use it, the practice-employed nurses and the attached nursing-staff or specified individuals?

(d) Interview-room

Often in a busy centre a small interview-room is a useful addition; it can sometimes act as an overflow consultation-room, or a consultation-room for the health visitor or midwife.

(e) Staff-rooms and Doctors' Common-room

The employment of additional staff by the practice inevitably means consideration of the need to provide a rest-room; sometimes a room (such as an interview-room) which can be used for more than one purpose might serve. In some practices doctors and staff may agree to share a common-room. If the centre is large enough then the common-room can double as the library.

To earn its place in the centre, the rest-room should encourage relaxation and friendly exchange of news and views amongst staff and doctors. Such a room does not have to be near the centre of the building, indeed it is often better if it is isolated from the main concourse so that it has the benefits of being both quiet and private away from patients using the rest of the building.

(f) The Special Needs of Teaching Practices

Special consideration must be given to the additional accommodation needed for teaching. The cost limits (see Chapter 4) make special allowances for practices where it is intended to undertake clinical teaching. The type of teaching is unspecified and might include both undergraduate training, vocational training and teaching members of professions allied to medicine. They allow the provision of slightly larger consulting-rooms and of a room for a trainee practitioner.

The special needs of a teaching practice include space for a small library, containing basic medical reference books and general practice medical journals. Some practices may wish to provide an audio-visual slide/tape unit for trainees to use with slides/tapes from the Graves Medical Audiovisual Library (formerly known as the Medical Recording Service Foundation).

4. Types of Premises

A growing number of doctors now work from purpose-built premises. These can be provided by the doctors themselves or rented either from an Area Health Authority (health centre) or a private landlord.

(a) Health Centres

The 1948 NHS Act envisaged the widespread provision of health centres by Local Health Authorities. For many reasons the health centre programme developed slowly, and only within the last ten years has it gained real momentum.

Since the reorganisation of the administrative structure of the NHS in 1974, responsibility for the provision and maintenance of health centres has been taken over by the Area Health Authorities (AHAs) which now rent accommodation in health centres to general practitioners.

The concept of a health centre was such that all the community services could be housed under one roof. Needless to say, few health centres provide all these services and the contemporary view is that each health centre should try to meet the needs of the local community.

Consequently, a health centre should provide accommodation for general practitioners and their staff, together with health service workers in associated fields such as community nursing sisters, health visitors and midwives—all those in fact who make up the primary health care team. In addition, space is usually set aside for providing those services which remain the responsibility of the AHA or Local Authority: the school health service, the chiropodist, some family planning clinics, children's clinics, and the child guidance service. In some centres it may be possible to provide facilities for a speech therapist, for an occupational therapist and for a physiotherapist. The closest co-operation of the primary health care team with others working in the community can be achieved if they are all based in the same building.

A good health centre should not be cramped for space. The need for a service in a community may develop and lack of accommodation can thwart its institution. A large room, basically for health education, can be adapted to provide all sorts of additional facilities. Many of these services may be provided independently by the Area Health Authority. Health centres are often built with separate general practitioner and community health sections.

However, if a general practitioner working in a health centre wishes to run any special clinics, then he is at liberty to do so. Indeed, many family doctors prefer to provide a developmental screening or family planning service as part of their ordinary consultation service, whilst others set aside specific time for such work.

The services which a general practitioner may provide from premises within a health centre are virtually unrestricted, though recently some Area Health Authorities have attempted to introduce some restrictions which the medical profession has successfully opposed. He has freedom to carry on private practice in conjunction with his NHS practice provided that this represents less than 50 per cent of his total practice income (subject to the usual abatements of reimbursement of rents and salaries of staff, if the private income earned in the health centre exceeds 10 per cent of his NHS income – Red Book para. 51.15).

A previously dispensing practitioner may elect to continue his dispensing service from the health centre and his accommodation would therefore include a dispensary.

It is clearly essential that the doctor thinking of moving into a health centre should be clear as to what his accommodation and staffing needs are likely to be, to discuss these with the Family Practitioner Committee (FPC) and AHA representative and to see that his rental contract covers all of them. Chapter 9 explains how the rental is calculated.

(b) Purpose-built Private Group Centres

Private group centres are usually provided by the general practitioner and his partners with the help of a mortgage. This may be arranged through the General Practice Finance Corporation or through a bank or building society. Less commonly, premises are built by a private land-lord (who may or may not be one of the partners) and rented to the group of doctors.

There is no reason why such purpose-built centres should not be at least as comprehensive in accommodation and design as the best health centres. The cost rent scheme (see Chapter 4) means that a doctor or group of doctors can finance all interest charges on a mortgage arranged through the General Practice Finance Corporation, by the notional rent (cost rent) received from the FPC.

(c) Adapted Premises

There will remain a large group of doctors who practise from existing rented or owner-occupied premises. Some of these may have provided medical services for many years. Often, whilst not clinically ideal, they may find favour with both the doctors and the patients for reasons of situation and convenience as well as sentiment. In some cases no reasonable alternative building or site may be available.

In owner-occupied premises the FPC will pay a notional rent which recognises the capital investment of the doctors in the premises. This rent is usually agreed in negotiation with the District Valuer. Where premises are rented, providing the rent is agreed to be 'fair' by the District Valuer, the FPC reimburses the rent. Doctors wishing to improve existing premises may apply for improvement grants of up to 30 per cent of the cost. Fuller details of this scheme are explained in the next chapter.

5. Branch Surgeries

Many practices have branch surgeries. The regulations governing the reimbursement of rent or payment of notional rent apply to branch surgeries as well as main surgeries. Doctors may obtain such payments in respect of all approved premises.

Often branch surgeries result from historical amalgamations of separate practices. They may be seen as providing for the convenience of patients isolated from the main centre of the practice. Some branch surgeries are little more than prescription collection centres, often without proper waiting-rooms or the facilities for the examination of patients. Some doctors feel that if such patients are really to benefit from the service of the branch surgery, then it should be no less well equipped and staffed than the central surgery. On the other hand, other doctors feel that half a loaf is better than none at all, and even relatively poorly equipped premises provide a place for consultation which might not otherwise take place.

Branch surgeries cause a duplication of services and complicate administration. The costs of such duplication must be set against possible financial gain from additional patients brought to the practice.

Table 3.1: Comparison between Health Centre and Owner-occupied Practice

	HEALTH CENTRE	OWNER-OCCUPIED PRACTICE CENTRE
1. Capital Financing	No problem for doctors. Provided by Area Health Authority (AHA).	Need for long-term financial planning and provision of capital at an early stage in a GP's career.
2. Capital Appreciation	Nil.	Long-term appreciation.
3. Changes in Buildings and Services	Negotiated through AHA. Although GPs working in the premises can influence the AHA, the approach to innovations may be rigid and facilities may become out-dated.	Under direct control of GPs system likely to be more flexible and adaptable to changing needs. (Occasionally an improvement grant may be claimed for capital expenditure on patient or staff facilities.)
4. Control of Use of Building	GP has no control on total use though may influence this through the local admin-istrative structure.	GP and partners have total control. They may invite other members of the primary health care team to suggest changes in building use.
5. Withdrawal from the NHS	The doctor would lose his right to practise from the health centre (though he is protected until suitable alternative accommodation is found).	Doctor would lose reimburse-ments of rent and rates, but not tenure of his premises.
6. Employment of Staff	Staff may be shared with AHA. Appointment may be by joint committee—potentially inflexible, disagreements between AHA and GPs pos-sible. GP does, however, have the right to employ his own staff.	Some staff may be employed by AHA, but the GP controls the appointment and dismissal of all other staff and directs their work (receptionists, secretaries, practice nurses). More flexibility possible.
7. Design	Standard design encouraged.	Personal variation encouraged.

In some ways, even if well equipped, branch surgeries are a potential hazard to patients since no one has yet planned a completely safe system which enables patients' records to be kept in more than one place at once (except possibly in those practices where records are computer held).

Doctors should attempt to evaluate the need for subsidiary premises and decide whether better care could equally or more efficiently be provided at the main centre. If a change in the policy of the practice towards branch surgeries is contemplated it is essential to discuss this with the Family Practitioner Committee. They will wish to be assured that the service to patients will not suffer before giving their consent to any changes. Local communities will frequently object to the closure of branch surgeries. Difficulties may be minimised if patients are fully informed beforehand about the reasons for the change and the arrangements for alternative care shown to be adequate. One main argument in favour of the continuance of small branch surgeries is the lack of adequate rural transport. Amongst the solutions which have been tried is the provision of a surgery minibus service which brings patients into the main centre where the facilities of properly equipped premises are available.

6. Comparisons between Health Centres and Owner-occupied Purpose-built Centres

It is difficult to compare the advantages and disadvantages of the two basic types of general practitioner accommodation. However, Table 3.1 lists differences under relevant headings. Basically, the advantages of the owner-occupied centre stem from the freedom of choice which the owner-doctor and his colleagues have, and the greater freedom to adapt their premises to changing conditions.

References and Further Reading

Forman, J.A.S. *Update Plus*, 1 (1971), pp. 265-70.
Jacka, S.M. & Griffiths, D.G. *Treatment-room Nursing* (Blackwell, 1976).
Practice in Health Centres (BMA, Scottish Office, 1977). This memorandum was prepared by a working group of the Scottish General Medical Services Committee for the guidance of general practitioners contemplating taking up practice in health centres.
Thomson, W.A.R., MD, ed. *The Doctor's Surgery* (The Practitioner Ltd, 1964). Although many of the problems described in this book were those facing general practitioners in the 1960s, the solutions are often still relevant today. It is a particularly valuable guide for practitioners wishing to plan or adapt their premises and organisation.

4 PREMISES: PLANNING AND IMPROVING

Few general practitioners are practising in premises which have remained
unchanged over the past twenty years. The changes may have been
relatively minor, or have involved major upheavals or a move to new
premises. We believe that practitioners are becoming more aware of
deficiencies in their premises and methods of working – and that most
general practitioners will at some time be involved in the financing and
design of improvements or premises which is the subject of this chapter.

1. Planning Purpose-built Premises

Although most doctors who join existing practices will not be involved
in planning new premises, all doctors should be aware of certain basic
considerations in the planning of purpose-built premises and an understanding of them will help the prospective partner assess the premises
from which he may be working.

Architects can give tremendous help to doctors designing premises,
but they need help themselves in understanding their clients' requirements. It is important to prepare a clear written brief, in which the
doctors list their needs, state reasons for them and indicate priorities.
The preparation of such a document by the partners will take time,
but should help them in thinking through the new pattern of work
which the new building may encourage. When a new element in primary
care is to be introduced, for example a treatment-room when the
doctors did not have one before, then the architect should know in
what way the existing work pattern of the doctors is expected to change
in the new building.

A second consideration is that everyone who expects to work in the
new building should be involved in the planning from an early stage.
Receptionists, secretaries, nurses, health visitors and practitioners have
different requirements and different priorities. Early consultation will
help minimise mistakes in design which may be costly or impossible to
correct after the building is completed.

Advice is available from various sources. The Central Information
Service for General Practice is an advisory service which is available to
all general practitioners in the United Kingdom. Its secretary may be

contacted at the Royal College of General Practitioners' headquarters. It has published a gazetteer of general practice which contains much practical advice. Visits to other practices, sometimes with staff or architect, are also extremely valuable as a way of crystallising ideas. Design points which are successful may be incorporated, unsuccessful design avoided.

(a) Health Centres: Special Points of Design and Financing

When a health centre is planned, all the general practitioners practising in the immediate area have a right to move into the new centre. Often the initiative in starting the process of designing and building a health centre comes from some of the local general practitioners themselves. At an early stage, all general practitioners in the area are notified of the intention to plan a health centre and are offered the use of its facilities. If a majority indicate support for a health centre then the project takes a step forward.

All those interested should have an opportunity of taking part in the planning decisions, and at least one of the general practitioners concerned will be appointed to the project planning committee. Thus, the general practitioners who will work in the building can have an important say in the design of the building. The more interest the doctors take in the planning the better the building is likely to be.

In large health centres there will almost certainly be Area Health Authority staff working in their own sections. For example, the senior nursing officer and the district community physician may have their offices there, and they themselves may have secretarial and administrative assistants. The district social services team may also be based in the same building. Such a centre increases the general practitioner's chances of meeting those working in other fields of community care and should be valued as an opportunity to reduce sectional barriers and improve the quality of care available to patients.

The doctor is expected to provide all his own practice equipment, whilst the authority will provide the standard fixtures. There can be a lot of disagreement over what is considered standard and what is extra. Equipment such as an electrocardiograph might be considered an extraordinary item, whereas wall-mounted sphygmomanometers might be standard. The AHA may agree to provide extra equipment and charge the doctor an annual fee for its lease.

There is another category of equipment which includes items which are shared. For example, if a treatment-room is used by the AHA Family Planning Clinic, then the provision of sterilisers and even specula might be considered as for joint use. In the same way, an audiometer would usually be needed for child developmental clinics but the AHA might agree that such items could be used by the general practitioners. There is no set rule about charges in these circumstances. They should be negotiated individually.

The payment which a general practitioner makes to the Area Health Authority for use of health centre premises consists of two elements. The first is rental for the premises themselves which is reimbursed. The second is a consolidated service charge (further discussed in Chapter 9). The service charges are deducted by the FPC from the quarterly payments made to practitioners. They constitute a business expense and should be charged against tax (Chapter 9). Although rent and reimbursement in most health centre practices is a book transaction at FPC level, it is essential for the correct calculation of practice expenses that the rent be declared as a practice expense in the practice accounts (see Appendix C).

(b) Private Purpose-built Centres: Special Points of Design and Financing

The same basic considerations of design apply equally to private purpose-built premises and health centres. In the former, the doctor is very much more involved for not only will he practise from the premises, but over the course of years he will become the owner of the freehold property. As such the building may more readily reflect the personalities of those working in it.

Many private purpose-built centres are financed by doctors, through a loan from the General Practice Finance Corporation. This is a government guaranteed body which raises money on the normal City of London money market. Consequently it varies its interest rate from time to time according to the standard market forces in operation at that moment. Loans are granted for a fixed term at a fixed rate of interest. Reimbursement of a notional rent by the appropriate Family Practitioner Committee (see Chapter 8) covers the interest payments for the loan in most cases. However, there are several points of practical importance.

(i) The effective rate for cost rent purposes is that rate of interest being charged at the time the doctor accepts a tender from a builder for the new purpose-built building, but the rate of interest charged by the Finance Corporation is that rate of interest currently in force at the time the doctor draws his first tranche of the loan. For example: if the loan is being sought at a time of rapidly varying money supply, rates of interest might change within months and the doctor could find himself with a fixed cost rent at, say, 16 per cent but an interest rate being charged by the Finance Corporation at, say, 17 per cent. (If he were fortunate, of course, interest rates might move in the opposite direction and he might find his cost rent being paid at a slightly higher rate than he was being charged on his loan.)

It is therefore important that solicitors and accountants involved in the arrangement of such a loan should be aware of these problems and wherever possible try to negotiate the acceptance of the tender and the drawing of the first tranche from the Finance Corporation at one and the same time. It is surprising how difficult it is to make such a co-ordinated arrangement, but most banks are prepared to make a bridging loan to doctors to meet initial expenses to allow the drawing of the first part of mortgage to coincide with the acceptance of a builder's tender.

(ii)   Another common problem which requires doctors to borrow money before they are ready to draw a mortgage from the General Practice Finance Corporation is that land purchase often precedes the acceptance of a builder's tender by many months. The security of the land is usually sufficient to guarantee a bank loan. If bank managers are not prepared to meet the doctors' loan requirements against such a security, other short-term loans might be raised by the doctors themselves through insurance companies. It is important to gain the Family Practitioner Committee's approval at the earliest possible stage to ensure that all allowable expenses may be claimed later.

(iii)   It is important to ensure that the Regional Medical Officer of the DHSS gives his approval to the design of the proposed premises. The design must meet the basic requirements laid down in the regulations concerning the cost rent scheme. If doctors build premises which do not meet those requirements, they may find that their cost rental will be affected. There are, incidentally, cost limits which are reviewed at regular intervals, but in a time of rapidly rising building prices it may be that a particular design cannot be built within these cost limits. If this is likely to be the case then the doctors and their architect should conduct negotiations with the Regional Medical Officer to see whether or not there is some special reason why costs are high (for example a difficult site) and to see whether a special cost limit for the project can be agreed. The need to seek agreement before work is started cannot be over-emphasised.

(iv)   Unfortunately, any doctor deciding to build his own purpose-designed premises will find that not only does he need to seek the approval of the health authorities in the guise of the Family Practitioner Committee and Regional Medical Officer, but he also has to satisfy the Local Authority Planning Department. His architect will obviously know how to go about this but occasionally the differing requirements of the two authorities may cause frustration for those not expecting problems.

(v) The doctor, or doctors, involved in the arrangement of the General Practice Finance Corporation loan will need to have some guarantee which they can offer the Corporation over the repayment of their mortgage. Such a guarantee must ensure repayment of the loan should the doctor die prematurely and also provide the capital sum due at the agreed term of the loan. It is usual to negotiate a loan for a period of 20-25 years.

In some cases the doctor undertakes to pay a set interest charge (deducted quarterly by the Family Practitioner Committee, and balanced by the monthly payments of notional rent) throughout the term of the loan. At the end of the term, the capital has to be paid back to the General Practice Finance Corporation. The provision of this capital sum usually requires the individual doctor to arrange some sort of linked life assurance or mortgage protection policy.

In other cases, the doctor undertakes to repay capital and interest (deducted quarterly by the Family Practitioner Committee) so that at the end of the term of the mortgage, the final repayment represents the last part of outstanding loan. With this type of repayment arrangement, there is still a need for insurance, but usually the cheaper mortgage protection type of policy will be sufficient.

Since the sums involved may be quite large, it is important to have skilled advice about the best type of insurance. Endowment assurances with profits may in the long run prove to be the most financially advantageous form, but, for the doctor who may possibly already be financing his own house purchase, the heavy premium payments may mean that some other type of insurance would be more appropriate.

Various insurance companies, including the Medical Sickness Society, have developed special types of policy which combine the traditional endowment assurance with profits with a reducing mortgage protection policy. These companies and most insurance brokers, accountants or bank managers can give advice on such matters, and the General Practice Finance Corporation itself may give helpful ideas to doctors using its service.

(vi) One further charge which the doctors must meet will be the expenses incurred in the day-to-day management of *their* building and the routine maintenance. These items would equate with the service charge made in health centres. Most organised practices will arrange a special account into which a regular sum is paid to underwrite unexpected expenses and redecoration.

(vii)   When a doctor joins a practice where there is an existing purpose-built surgery already financed by a loan from the General Practice Finance Corporation there may be problems. These arise usually because the retiring general practitioner or the existing partners require the incoming partner to take a share in the financial responsibility for the freehold property. In this case, the new doctor will be faced both with the possible purchase of his own house and the responsibility of raising a large sum of money to buy into the freehold of the partnership's premises. Most partnerships will try to make this as easy as possible for their new partner but, in spite of this, his initial reaction may be one of fright when he looks at his total borrowing requirements. Nevertheless, he should understand that as far as the practice premises are concerned, he can borrow directly from the General Practice Finance Corporation at their current rate of interest. The conditions of the loan are similar to those described above for doctors building their own premises except that he will have to pay the current rate to the Finance Corporation. New arrangements are currently (1980) being negotiated between the profession (GMSC) and the DHSS to enable the new partner to claim an increased cost rental payment if his interest rate payable to the General Practice Finance Corporation is higher than that paid by the existing partners on their borrowing.

(viii)   Paying off the General Practice Finance Corporation and other loans by partnerships is a very complicated affair, especially if the doctors in the partnerships are drawing different percentages of the partnership profits. Some accountants with experience in such matters adjust the capital accounts of each partner annually to balance changes in the assets of the partnership produced by quarterly repayments of capital to the General Practice Finance Corporation.

(c) Premises Rented from Independent Landlords: Special Points of Financing

In the case of premises provided by an independent landlord, if they have been purpose-built for the doctors concerned, it is essential that agreement should be reached with the Family Practitioner Committee that the cost rent scheme is applicable before the doctor is committed to renting the premises. The same requirements regarding cost limits will apply if the full rental charge by the landlord is to be refunded as a cost rental from the Family Practitioner Committee. There are some advantages to the system of a private landlord providing premises for a group of doctors. For example, it may be that one or more doctors in a partnership are prepared to finance the premises for the whole partnership, and that the other partners do not wish to be involved in raising money through a mortgage but are prepared to pay a rent for the provision of premises. However, such an arrangement does preclude the non-freeholders from the security provided by property ownership, and from the possibility of a long-term gain in the capital value of the premises in which they work.

2. Improvement of Existing Premises

As the demands made upon a medical practice change, so the doctors may agree that certain improvements in the existing premises are necessary to cover the requirements. Where improvements are to be made to facilities used by patients or staff, then the Department of Health and Social Security is able to make an improvement grant of up to 30 per cent of the cost of the work. Such grants are not payable for accommodation used primarily by the doctors (including consulting-rooms and doctors' common-rooms).

In order to agree an improvement grant, it is necessary first to be clear in one's own mind and the minds of partners, which improvements are necessary to the practice. Most doctors will need to employ the services of an architect. Before committing themselves to any major expenditure, they should seek the advice of the Family Practitioner Committee, since no improvement grant may be claimed if work has been started on the project before agreement with the FPC has been reached. The Committee itself is only authorised to agree to improvements costing up to a limit of £2,050 (1980). Applications involving larger sums have to be submitted to the DHSS through the FPC. The maximum grant per practitioner is £4,100 and there is an overall limit of grant of £14,350 per project (1980).

The present arrangements for improvement grants are flexible so that a mixed scheme may be developed. Practitioners who wish to improve their existing premises may do so partly through the cost rent scheme and partly with the help of an improvement grant. With such an arrangement the initial net capital outlay may be reduced.

Further Reading

Department of Health and Social Security. *Health Centres: A Design Guide*

(Welsh Office: HMSO, 1970).

Scottish Home and Health Department. *Design Guide: Health Centres in Scotland* (London: HMSO, 1973).

5 RECEPTION: THE 'SHOP FRONT'

The initial impression gained by a patient when he enters his doctor's premises is most important. He or she may base future expectations of the practice on their first impressions and this may affect the process of the consultation. How often does one hear the comment, 'I couldn't get an appointment with my doctor for five days,' or 'His waiting-room is cold,' or 'The only reading material is four-year-old copies of *Punch* and *Tatler*!'

With the financial help which general practitioners now obtain for staff, rent, rates and running costs of premises, there is no excuse for the old 'lock up' type surgery with lino on the floor, dreary lines of hard chairs and a doctor who has so few staff that he is constantly interrupted by the telephone during his consultations.

When planning his practice the doctor should pay great attention to his reception area, waiting-room and staff as in the long run this will certainly contribute more to his professional reputation in the eyes of most of the patients than any number of medical qualifications.

The Reception Area

When a patient walks into the surgery premises it should be immediately apparent where he should report his arrival. The reception desk should be clearly labelled with the doctor's name, particularly in practices where the premises may be large with several practitioners or groups operating from them. The desk itself should be about three-and-a-half feet high and twelve inches wide so that the patient can lean comfortably on it but not over it. Behind the desk should be a wide shelf on which rests the appointment book.

Often the receptionist will have to ask the patient questions which may be confidential and so attention should be paid to this in the design. Confidentiality can be helped by individual reception booths, well screened from the waiting area.

The noise in the reception area should be kept to a minimum. Telephones, for example, can be of the trimphone variety and tuned to the soft tone which is less intrusive than the harsh clamour of a bell. If at all possible, secretarial and typing work should be done in a separate office.

The Waiting Room

This should be comfortable, light and airy with some form of carpeting
to reduce noise. Many of the nylon tiles now on sale are very hard
wearing and not particularly expensive. The furniture may be of assorted
shapes with a fair proportion of upright chairs which can be moved
around or stored if not in use. A number of quite comfortable stacking
chairs are available. If possible, there should be some easy chairs with
hard-wearing nylon covers to enable them to be wiped down easily.
The number of chairs in a waiting-room is a matter of personal taste,
but an efficient appointment system allows a reduction in the number
required. Five chairs for each doctor consulting is a suggested figure.

Many purpose-built premises incorporate a children's room along-
side the waiting-room with reinforced glass doors which enable mothers
and staff to keep an eye on what is happening inside. Putting child-
sized tables and chairs in a room of this sort with an assortment of robust
toys will keep young children much happier while waiting to see the
doctor than fidgeting on a hard chair with nothing to do.

The waiting area should ideally be placed in a position to be
directly supervised by the reception staff. If it is possible to have a
sliding glass window overlooking the waiting-room then this solves the
problem and prevents conversation in the office from being overheard.

Pictures on the walls of the waiting-room are always appreciated.
Exhibitions of a local art society are often particularly interesting and
can be sold to benefit their funds. Schools may be pleased to contribute children's work and these simple measures give the patients
further topics to distract them and something to discuss and criticise
other than the doctors!

The Appointment System

During the last ten years many practices have introduced appointment
systems. The reasons for not having them include:

(1) Personal resistance on the part of senior doctors who have always
had an open surgery.
(2) Rural areas where surgery attendances have to be geared to
infrequent buses and other problems of transport.
(3) Small branch surgeries where small numbers of patients and few
or no staff make appointments impracticable.

(4) Inability to maintain a flexible system.

However, for the majority of patients and doctors a well-organised appointment system has made life much pleasanter. Some advantages of a well-run appointment system are:

(1) Less waiting for the patients.

(2) The ability to make the full use of consulting-rooms throughout the day, particularly when two doctors have to use one room.

(3) The more efficient use of doctor time and the ability to direct the workload to periods of the day when it fits in with his timetable.

(4) Because the patient knows that he will not have a long wait in a crowded room he is more willing to come to surgery with a condition for which otherwise he might request a visit.

(5) The practice nurse can have advance warning of the consultations in which she will be involved during the doctor's surgery (such as repeat pill checks).

(6) If one particular doctor is getting heavily overbooked the tactful use of an appointment system can be used to direct patients to another doctor who is not so busy, if this is the agreed practice policy.

(7) Urgent consultations and children with infectious illness, such as rubella, can be seen between routine appointments by using a side room and the practice nurse to receive them.

(8) Doctors with appointment systems tend to spend longer with their patients in each consultation.

(9) Less space is required in the waiting-room.

(10) Follow-up consultations may be arranged around a doctor's holidays or study leave so that continuity of supervision may be more readily maintained.

Some disadvantages are:

(1) Appointment systems which are overloaded for one reason or another will result in patients being told that they cannot see the doctor for several days. This is unrealistic and is not the fault of the appointment system but of the organisation behind it, which should be flexible enough to deal with extra patient demand as well as unexpected emergencies.

(2) Some patients are incapable of making appointments for one reason or another and prefer to 'drop in'.

(3) Running an appointment system does mean that more staff have to be employed to answer the telephone to make appointments. There is, therefore, an increased expenditure on salaries.
(4) Staff need special training in managing an appointment system.
(5) The elderly and women with large families often find it difficult to organise themselves to fit in with their appointment time.

The Lloyd-Hamol appointment book with loose leaf pages is now in popular use and is very flexible. When the doctor is deciding about his surgery times and appointments a number of factors should be borne in mind:

1. His rate of consultation.
2. The time he has available for consultation.
3. Other demands upon his room if he is sharing it.
4. Re-booking of patients.

These four factors will now be discussed in detail.

1. The Rate of Consultation

Some doctors take a pride in seeing large numbers of patients in the shortest time possible, but this attitude does not make for the good practice of medicine or patient satisfaction.

Probably a satisfactory rate is about eight patients per hour except in times of unusual and extreme pressure. A booking of six per hour should perhaps be a reasonable target. It is vital that patients contacting the surgery at a reasonably early hour should be able to get an appointment that day, if requested, with the doctor of their choice as often as possible. In determining the priority of the booking, patients should not have to be subjected to 'third degree' by the receptionist. Bad feeling created by the receptionist often carries over into the consultation with the doctor.

Some practices find that a satisfactory method is to book at not less than ten minute intervals up until the day concerned. Spaces may then be left, perhaps two spaces on each hour and half-hour for extra emergency bookings. This system has the advantages of providing space for patients who wish to be seen the same day and also provides a few excess patients who can be seen if someone fails to turn up or is late.

2. The Time Available for Consultation

Many doctors adhere rigidly to the old 9-10.30 a.m. and 5-6 p.m.
regime. If they do this their appointment system is doomed to failure.
The whole essence must be flexibility. If the demand is such then the
doctor must be prepared to go on for an extra hour or so at each
session. It will certainly be repaid many times over by a decrease in
patients requesting visits because they were unable to get an appointment and a decrease in the incidence of late night calls for patients
who were stalled by the receptionist until the following day. A
suggested time for surgeries would be, therefore, something like 9-11.30
a.m. and 4-6 p.m. depending on local and individual circumstances.

Some doctors still run their afternoon surgeries well on into the
evening because they start them far too late. Occasionally a man
at work will be unable to get away early but this is becoming
increasingly rare and the last few appointments of the day can be
kept for just such a situation.

There is still a strong resistance to running afternoon sessions from
2 p.m. but this should be considered if space is at a premium in the
premises. Many patients, for example mothers with families, like to
come at this time of day.

3. Other Demands on His Room

If a doctor has to share his consulting-room with someone else it poses
a number of problems. The irritation can be reduced to a minimum by
making sure that there is at least half-an-hour between the last appointment of the first surgery and the first appointment of the following
surgery, but we feel that sharing a consulting-room is a potent cause of
irritation between doctors. In addition, it makes it much more difficult
for the room to reflect the personality of either doctor.

4. Re-booking of Patients

One of the main reasons why patients asking for an appointment to see
their doctor are told that they cannot have one for several days is
because he is fully booked with follow-up cases. Of course many
patients will have to be recalled at intervals for all sorts of reasons.
However, if one doctor finds himself constantly booked up far ahead

compared with his partners then he should reappraise his recall criteria. A doctor should be clear in his own mind why he is asking a patient to return to see him. It may be for reasons concerned with routine surveillance in hypertension, for example; it may be because he is unsure of the diagnosis and wishes to check again or it may be to see that his treatment has worked. New entrants to general practice tend to ask patients to return more often because of their inexperience of the natural history of disease and their lack of confidence in their own ability.

If a patient tells the receptionist that he has to make an appointment for a month ahead, the receptionist should be encouraged to use her discretion about the actual day booked for that appointment. If four weeks to the day is already getting booked up or the doctor has other extra demands on that particular day, then she could make the appointment for one of several days either side of the suggested date. Doctors can greatly help their receptionists by not specifying an exact day but saying, 'Please make an appointment in about a month.'

If all these factors are considered when organising appointments, most systems should run smoothly except for unforeseen occasions, such as an influenza epidemic or the doctor being unexpectedly called away. This brings up the important point of punctuality. If a doctor expects his patients to arrive punctually for their appointments, then he should start his surgery on time. It is no good regularly starting half-an-hour late and wondering why your appointment system does not work.

From time to time it is worth carrying out a simple check on the system by asking patients at random how long they had to wait (a) for an appointment and (b) in the surgery that day. If the answer to these questions is frequently more than 24 hours or 15 minutes respectively, then the doctor should review his appointment system.

The Call System

A patient has to be informed that the doctor is ready to see him and there are several ways in which this can be done.
(1) *In person.* The doctor may come to the door and call the next patient. This has the personal touch but can be time-consuming and also tiring to do twenty times during a surgery.
(2) *The intercom system.* There are several systems available and it is a good precaution to invest in the best that the doctor can afford.

Some of the cheap ones break down quickly and are so unintelligible as to be useless. The doctor can either call reception on the intercom and ask for the next patient to be sent or speak directly to the waiting-room. The disadvantage of the latter is that deaf or elderly patients may mishear instructions or there may be three 'Mrs Smiths' sitting there. Patients prefer to be called personally if this is at all possible, and a good receptionist can be as welcoming as the doctor himself.

(3) *A buzzer or light system.* A simple buzzer and light system can be used. When the doctor presses a switch a light comes on beside the name and a buzzer sounds. The light may be situated in the reception and the staff then send the next patient in or it may be situated in the waiting-room. The disadvantage of the latter is that the patients may not know who is next unless they have also been issued with a numbered disc as they arrived.

(4) The more elaborate methods described in (2) and (3) are almost certainly required if an appointment system is in operation and the reception staff will need to know who has arrived and who is next due to see the doctor. If there is no appointment system then just giving the patient a number as he arrives may be all that is needed to ensure a smooth flow of patients, each one going in to see the doctor as the last one leaves, but it does lack the personal touch.

The Telephone System

The larger the premises the more complex will be the GPO system used. The Post Office can provide small switchboards with two or three external lines and six to twelve internal extensions to large private automatic exchanges with many external lines and multiple internal extensions. The more complex the system the more necessary it is to have staff specifically trained in its use. The Post Office will train staff to use the equipment and ex-GPO telephone operators can often be usefully employed as switchboard operators/receptionists.

The telephone cover for out-of-hours must be considered when installing equipment, with the following possibilities:

(1) If all partners live within a mile of the central surgery then the provision of external extensions to their homes may be practicable. The charge for this depends on the distance involved but at present (1980) a line of one kilometre would mean a £50 connection charge and £20 per quarter rental. The partner will have to have two telephones in his

house, one being a surgery extension and one an outside line or else he will have to have a special telephone with an attachment which enables him to be switched through to the extension.

(2) For doctors living some distance from the surgery premises, an interception system will have to be considered.

(a) The Post Office charges for intercepting a call and re-routing it are now very high (35p per change of transfer in 1980).

(b) It is possible to rent from the GPO an answering device which can make a statement lasting 20 seconds or 90 seconds. The rent paid is double for the instrument which gives the longer time. In fact, the 20 second record is quite sufficient to leave a message such as, 'The surgery is now closed. If you require a doctor in emergency please phone Dr X at . . .' It is essential that the message should be spoken slowly and with clarity. The message automatically repeats itself after 20 seconds and so the whole of the time should be used for the message otherwise the caller may replace the receiver before the repeat.

(c) The commercial answering machines have the advantage of the caller being able to record a message if required but have the disadvantage of being quite expensive and there is usually a long rental lease.

(3) A further interception method is the subscriber transfer system for individuals of groups. By this method a central switchboard line can be re-routed to another external number automatically. In addition it is possible by dialling codes to transfer the calls from one extension number to another without returning to the central switchboard. This has the advantage for a group of doctors of providing a method of putting the duty line through to the appropriate person who can then later transfer it to someone else or to a 'telephone minder' when his duty is completed. Transfers can only be made between lines previously linked in the system by the Post Office. The equipment involved is expensive to install and rent, and is not always available if sub-station telephone exchanges are involved. The current prices can be obtained from the Post Office Sales Department.

(4) A resident caretaker may take all calls and pass them on to the duty doctor.

(5) A deputising service may be used when all calls are intercepted by operator or ansaphone and re-routed to this service.

A practice must decide which system suits its arrangements best and arrange its telephone system accordingly. The doctor should always

bear in mind that he has a responsibility to provide 24-hour cover for
his patients and he should ensure that the system used provides a
reasonable and reliable service for them.

The Medical Records

Medical record cards take up a great deal of space. Careful thought must
be given to the most appropriate method of storage depending on the
area available. The long-awaited arrival of A4 size records seems to be
indefinitely delayed but practices which use this size have even more of
a storage problem than others with the bulging FP 5/6 envelopes.
Storage systems are as follows:

(1) Lateral filing uses shelves to store records. This has the advantage
of easy access but care must be taken to avoid using shelves too high or
low for the staff to reach them, or a good step-up stool must be provided.
Remploy make a lateral file which can be simply adapted from FP 5/6
envelopes to A4 size wallets.

(2) Rotating systems. Several sizes of rotating drum are available
taking from 5,000-9,000 record cards. These drums have the advantage
of occupying less space in the office. The receptionist can stand and
rotate the drum thus avoiding unnecessary movement about the office.
It is possible to provide covers for these drums to make them secure.
The disadvantage is that they cost more than shelves or metal cabinets.

(3) Metal cabinets with drawers are commonly used. These have
the advantage of being robust and can be locked. The disadvantages are
that it is possible to tip them over if several top drawers are open
simultaneously (unless they are attached to the wall), drawers tend to
stick and are heavy for female staff to handle. Individual record cards
may be difficult to find if a drawer is tightly packed.

(4) Computer storage systems. Several areas of the country are
experimenting with the use of computers in general practice. These
systems are expensive in terms of capital expenditure but, once
installed, occupy much less space. One sheet of 6 in x 4 in microfiche
can hold 200 summarised records.

Staff

The staff who are present in the reception area, their attitude, knowledge and efficiency, are as important, if not more important, than the physical arrangements of the reception area itself. Their relationship with both patients and the doctors with whom they work determines to a large extent whether the practice runs smoothly from day to day or whether it lurches from crisis to crisis. The contracts which general practitioners have with their staff are fully discussed in Chapter 11, the financial arrangements concerning reimbursement and PAYE are described in the chapter on practice expenses (Chapter 9), and the philosophy behind the relationship and 'management' of staff within the practice are considered in Chapter 7.

In our opinion these questions are of prime importance. The success or failure of any organisation depends on the people who run it.

Further Reading

Drury, M. *The Medical Secretary's Handbook*, 3rd edition (London: Baillière Tindall, 1975).
Owen, H. *Administration in General Practice* (London: E. Arnold, 1975).

PART THREE: PEOPLE

6 TEAMWORK

History

The concept of the general-practice team developed only slowly. Certainly until the middle of the twentieth century the most common form of practice was that of a single doctor working, often with his wife to help him as secretary, with minimal or even no supporting staff at all. The doctor usually worked from his own house. District nurses and midwives worked in a district (employed initially by voluntary bodies, more recently by the Local Authority) and were not connected formally with practices in any way.

The first supporting staff to be recruited were receptionists followed in quick succession by secretaries. A few practices employed nurses but from the mid-1960s district nurses and health visitors were increasingly 'attached' or seconded to general practices by Local Authorities. By the mid-1970s about 70 per cent of such staff were attached. Since reorganisation of the NHS in 1974 district nurses and health visitors have been employees of the Area Health Authority rather than the Local Authority.

The so-called organisational revolution in general practice was pioneered by some practices in the 1950s and became widespread in the 1960s. Much of the early work and development was done by the Practice Organisation Committee of the Royal College of General Practitioners. The cost to general practices of employing nurses in practice was greatly reduced in 1966 by the charter for general practice negotiated between the then government and the BMA. This led to the introduction of reimbursement of 70 per cent of the salaries of approved staff to the limit of two full-time staff for each established principal.

The Team

Working in teams has both advantages and disadvantages. When considering the roles of the professional members of the team it is worth analysing some of the main principles of teamwork:

(1) Pooling

(2) Delegation
(3) Specialisation of function
(4) Multi-disciplinary discussion

(1) Pooling

Pooling is a form of teamwork in which two or more individuals co-operate in order to share a facility or service. It does not necessarily involve financial partnership and may or may not involve financial exchange. Its aims are primarily economic and administrative. The commonest example of pooling is where two or more professionals share both a building and secretarial services, as occurs when consultants share private rooms or when two or more general practitioners or partnerships share a common building. In the case of general practitioners the group practice allowance is a further inducement to share facilities. Such an arrangement may enable a group to afford equipment or additional staff.

Another example of this kind of working arrangement is the out-of-hours duty rotas operated by most general practitioners in Britain in which practitioners take it in turns to be on call for several colleagues in one or more practices.

(2) Delegation

A second aspect of medical teamwork is delegation, whereby someone is trained to perform work which would otherwise be done by the doctor. Delegation becomes cost effective when there is a saving of the doctor's time which, it is assumed, will be used for work which only a doctor can perform. Delegation ceases to be cost effective if the doctor does not make efficient use of the time saved. Delegated work remains the responsibility of the doctor, who has a legal and professional duty to satisfy himself of his staff's competence.

Common examples of this kind of delegation are receiving patients, filing, telephone answering, and some nursing procedures. The assumption is that this is work which the doctor could equally do himself or herself but chooses to delegate.

(3) Specialisation of Function (Division of Labour)

The third principle is that the team may include an individual who has a special skill or experience which is not otherwise available to a member of the existing team. When health visitors, for example, were first attached to general practices they brought with them to the teams they joined special experience and skill in advising about child-

rearing, in a systematic approach to preventive medicine and in case-
finding, which were generally absent from general practice at that time.
They retain today in most practices more skill in dealing with feeding
and many other child management problems than other members of
the team.

Similarly the secretaries, by bringing specific typing and dictating
skills to general practice, raised standards of communication (typed
letters and filed carbon copies) which could not be done by many
doctors themselves.

However, in general, division of labour becomes economic and
efficient only if the individual with the special skills uses them exclusively
or for most of his or her time.

(4) Discussion Between Colleagues

The most complex and perhaps the most exciting aspect of teamwork
is the discussion by colleagues of the problems of their work. The
concept of mutual co-operation between colleagues who are prepared
to discuss their work and the policies of the team is relatively new.
Few so far are prepared to give and take constructive criticism between
themselves.

Normally such exchanges will take place only if members of the
team feel secure and are on a par with one another. A hierarchy of rank
inhibits criticism as inferiors always hesitate to criticise their superiors.
Its potential in British general practice is thus at present mainly between
partners and colleagues in selected professions, such as health visitors
and nurses. The realisation of the concept depends on mutual trust
and a genuine willingness to consider new ideas and to adapt policy
through constructive criticisms.

Ideally the practice policies which are described elsewhere should
emerge from discussions of this kind and should have been well and
truly thrashed out in team discussion and be acceptable to all. Some
examples from our practices are given in Appendix B. Similarly the
feedback information described in Chapter 7 is a necessary precondition
for the review of policies and for the provision of a factual basis for
regular discussion. The organisation for such discussion will obviously
vary from practice to practice. Many find a weekly working lunch
suitable, others prefer evening meetings and yet others prefer group
discussion over coffee. The time and the setting matters little; the
personal relationships and the willingness to make constructive
criticism over the years is the key to progress. One measurement of the
success of such relationships is to ask periodically, 'What new service

is our team providing for patients which is measurably better than we did this time last year?'

The Disadvantages of Teamwork

So much is written about teamwork nowadays that it is easy to become complacent about its value. However, like all other systems of organisation and patterns of arrangement, it has its own disadvantages and adverse effects. These need to be considered as the efficiency of every team should be reviewed periodically by the members themselves, who should seek to measure the adverse effects of their own system and do what they can to minimise them.

1. Collusion of Anonymity

Balint, in his classic book *The Doctor, His Patient and the Illness*, introduced the idea of the 'collusion of anonymity', by which he meant that it was sometimes possible for a patient to become lost between different professionals all of whom were apparently dealing with him. This was because no single professional was accepting personal continuing responsibility for the patient.

Such collusion of anonymity easily occurs in practices still and needs to be identified by the members of the team as soon as possible. Having one named partner for each particular patient helps because health visitors, practice nurses and secretaries all know where responsibility lies. Where this is not done it becomes necessary for partners to agree regularly which doctor is accepting final responsibility. At times it is also necessary to agree responsibilities between health visitor colleagues and nurses.

2. Difficulties in Communication

The problems of difficulties in communication are discussed in Chapter 7. Good management must be designed to promote good communications. Lamberts & Riphagen (1975) have given examples of just how complex and difficult it can be to develop teamwork in general practice. It usually takes several years.

3. Time for Meetings

In practices which make a genuine attempt to promote communication and avoid the isolation of the members of the team, regular meetings are always necessary. These meetings may simply be 10 or 15 minute sessions in which two or more people meet together to discuss day-to-day problems and plans, or they may be more formal meetings, such as quarterly staff meetings for all members of the practice team.

The time these meetings take, however, needs to be monitored and assessed because they can take up too much time and may begin to encroach on the time available for patients. For example, in one of our practices the regular timetable each week includes on average two hours with the partners, a further two hours alone with the vocational trainee, an additional 1½ hours per week with the practice manager, the health visitor, the district nurse, and the doctors' secretary. This total of 5½ hours is equivalent, at an average consulting rate of eight patients per hour, to 44 consultations per week. In other words, the time spent each week in discussing the work of the team has been allocated a higher priority than seeing an additional 44 patients.

This balance of team discussion is about right only if useful discussions and decisions ensue. Work in a particular practice needs constant review, because the trend over the years seems always to be to increase the amount of discussion time at the expense of consulting time.

Similar problems can be seen in big hierarchical organisations, including other parts of the National Health Service. The danger of more complex medical organisations is that they start becoming increasingly bureaucratic to the detriment of the patient and client. This is an example of Parkinson's Law, i.e. 'Work expands to fill the time available'.

It is necessary somehow to ensure that the professionals do not just chat and that they really do use the time available together for improving policies for the care of patients by sharing information and consciously trying to plan a strategy for measuring standards of care and seeking to improve them.

The Members of the Team

There are three kinds of nurses who work in general-practice teams: health visitors, district nurses, and practice nurses. In addition most practices have attached midwives. All these professionals have separate skills which overlap. In particular they work in the patients' 'territory' – the home (Gray, 1978).

1. Health Visitors

Health visitors are always State Registered Nurses and usually State

Certified Midwives, although some only hold Part I of the SCM
Certificate. They also hold in addition the Health Visitors' Certificate
of the Council for the Education and Training of Health Visitors. The
regulations required of health visitors include statutory responsibilities,
i.e. laid down by Act of Parliament. The Health Visitors' Certificate is
now obligatory. In Britain there are about 8,000 health visitors, less
than half as many as general practitioners. The Department of Health
and Social Security recommends one health visitor for 4,500 patients.

Health visitors are employed by Health Authorities, and their management structure is part of that of the nursing profession as a whole. They
are immediately responsible to Nursing Officers and through them to
Community Nursing Officers to District Nursing Officers and ultimately
to the Area Nursing Officer of the Area Health Authority.

The role of the health visitor is:

(1) Home visiting. She is required to visit infants as soon as possible
after the midwife ceases to attend. This is usually between 10 and 28
days. Thereafter these visits are made regularly, especially during the
first year, until the child attends school.

(2) Clinic duties. Most health visitors are still required to attend health
authority clinics which are the successors to the infant welfare clinics.
There they have opportunities of advising about child care and feeding
and carrying out developmental assessments in association with health
authority doctors.

Increasingly these advisory and assessment functions are being taken
over by general practice. More and more practices are organising their
own well-baby clinics, either shared between the partners, held by one
partner on behalf of the practice, or more commonly, each doctor
seeing each child registered on his own list.

(3) Control of infectious diseases. Health visitors are concerned with
the personal and clinical aspects of infectious diseases and work with
general practitioners and when necessary with community physicians to
help to prevent the spread of such diseases in the community.

(4) Health education. Every contact between a health visitor and a
patient should be an opportunity for health education. Talks on child
care and hygiene to groups of mothers, help with health education
displays, encouragement to voluntary organisations are examples of
her methods.

(5) Social advice. Health visitors function in many practices as a source
of information and of the provision of reports, a role very similar in
many ways to that of social workers. The health visitor is often the link

between many general practices and social work departments of Local Authorities. This role may well change with the growing trend towards the attachment of social workers themselves to general practice.

Three-quarters of all health visitors in Great Britain are now attached to general practitioners and it is the policy of the Royal College of General Practitioners that this proportion should continue to increase.

2. District Nurses

District nurses are State Registered Nurses most of whom have taken an additional course in district nursing. They are employed by NHS health authorities and about three-quarters are now 'attached', i.e. seconded to general practitioners. They may work whole time or part time.

District nurses are perhaps the oldest and closest professional colleagues for general practitioners. They have a long history of caring for the sick in their own homes and their reputation among patients is usually very high. They have the extremely responsible job of providing all general nursing care in patients' homes. They have to work alone and largely unsupervised in a wide variety of conditions. It is the district nurse who does all the main nursing procedures for patients at home. These include temperature, pulse recording, giving injections, taking blood, ear syringing and dressings. In recent years district nurses have acquired more equipment such as ripple beds, and they can call on other services, such as bath attendants, night sitters, and soiled linen services.

They are experienced in helping families manage all types of sick people from those with incontinence to those with coronaries. They spend a large proportion of their time with the elderly (Harris & Jones, 1977) and are the key members of the health care team in the care of the dying at home.

The Queens Nursing Institute has recently (1979) issued a revised version of its booklet *Nursing in the Community* which describes in more detail the role and activities of community nurses.

3. The Practice Nurses

The practice nurse may be either a State Registered Nurse or State Enrolled. Because of the growing responsibilities of work in the treatment-room and potential difficulties with medico-legal complications, we recommend that general practitioners should usually employ State Registered Nurses. We advise that they be members of the Royal College of Nursing and thus covered by its indemnity scheme. The nurse's subscription can be added to her salary and reimbursement of the increased salary is then possible.

The role of the treatment-room sister or practice sister will vary from practice to practice and will largely depend on her interest and training, and the facilities available to her in her treatment-room. We regard the presence of a treatment-room as highly desirable in every modern general practice and its equipment is further described in Chapter 3. We recommend the title of 'practice sister' because this is work involving responsibility comparable to that of a ward sister in hospital. We believe that this work should be rewarded with sisters' pay. This work is particularly suitable for experienced nurses, especially those married with children who may be attracted by the possibility of part-time work. Many general practitioners have SRNs as patients who may be suitable for such posts.

The work of the treatment-room sister in a typical general practice is as follows:

Taking blood for investigations.
Dressings. Removal of sutures.
Injections: (a) therapeutic, e.g. antibiotics and vitamin replacement therapy, e.g. B12; (b) preventive, e.g. desensitisation.
Immunisations and vaccinations (except smallpox).
Treating warts.
Assisting the doctors with medical examinations, for example testing the urine, measuring the height, weight, visual acuity, colour vision, and blood pressure.
Ear syringing.
Following up selected groups of patients in the practice, especially those with hypertension, postgastrectomy, obesity, anaemia, schizophrenia, or patients on systemic steroids.
Controlling the stock in the treatment-room, re-ordering as necessary.
Maintaining the emergency treatment stock, taking blood, and assisting doctors in fitting intra-uterine devices.
Tine testing (Mantoux).

In Appendix C the practice nurse workload over the past four years of one of our practices, where three part-time SRNs work for a total of 32 hours with a population of 6,500 patients, is listed.

In other practices, sisters perform peak flow tests, geriatric checks, ECG tracing, pill checks, and cervical smears. A growing number of practice sisters are now undertaking contraceptive training and courses for this are available in most regions.

The principle is that doctors as employers have a legal and professional

duty to establish that the sister is competent and has been fully trained
to satisfactory standards. It is necessary to agree with the sister, as a
fellow professional, the guidelines of her work and to agree when referral
to doctors is expected, but also to work towards promoting the nurse's
autonomy, giving her as much clinical responsibility as she seeks and is
able to tolerate.

We believe that it is important to work towards a system where a
treatment-room sister is available to patients at the same time as a
doctor is holding a surgery. Whether or not the sister should be directly
accessible to the patients is a matter for each practice to decide but most
practices believe that an experienced sister should be available directly
since she can often deal herself with problems such as bites, stings, or
lacerations, and at the same time give much health education to the
patients she sees.

Fees

One of the difficulties in many areas is that Health Authority nursing
officers object to their staff carrying out work which entitles general
practitioners to item-of-service fees. We believe these feelings are due to
a misunderstanding of the mechanics of a doctor's remuneration. Unless
understood they may be a source of resentment. In some parts of Devon,
for example, Health Authority staff have been given instructions that
they shall not carry out any health procedures which will attract a fee
for the practice. This leads to the paradoxical situation that certain
treatments can be done while others cannot. It is clearly inefficient to
have highly qualified professionals in such a situation. The advantages
of the practice employing its own sister are obvious and this is happening
increasingly all over the country.

We believe the treatment-room should pay its way. Every treatment-
room should have a record of the procedures undertaken and this should
include the fees. An efficient nursing team should generate enough item-
of-service fees to cover at least the 30 per cent of their salaries which is
not directly reimbursed by the NHS. We do not feel that either doctors
or nurses should feel embarrassed about this; on the contrary it is good
preventive medicine and good practice organisation. Good practices are
often characterised by cost consciousness in prescribing, and have a
sensitive awareness of the cost of medical services. The same should
apply to nurses who are members of the team since it is government
policy that rubella, tetanus and polio immunisation, for example, should
be provided as a matter of public policy. The practice sister is ideally
placed to fulfil this government aim.

In general the potential role of the treatment-room nurse is relatively unfulfilled at present in general practice. However, it is likely to be developed substantially in the next few years (Bolden & Morgan, 1975).

4. Midwives

Few practices will be large enough to justify the attachment of a full-time midwife. The usual arrangements, therefore, are that the Health Authority employed midwife calls in at the practice on the days of the various antenatal clinics of the doctors and sees the patients in the doctors' practice at that time. These midwives normally visit at home as well and take part in the domiciliary midwifery service. This inevitably makes a close working relationship more difficult but since the same midwife is at all the antenatal clinics in a practice it is possible in time for her and the partners to get to know each other well enough to achieve a good teamwork relationship.

5. Social Workers

Social workers are not often attached to general practice although many are now working primarily in general practice, and a great many more have part-time liaisons of various kinds with a growing number of practices. Most social workers are employed not by the Health Authorities but by Local Authorities through Social Services Departments. A few may be privately sponsored through grants (Forman & Fairbairn, 1968; Paine, 1976). We recommend two books on the subject, Forman & Fairbairn (1968) and Goldberg & Neil (1972), to describe the pros and cons of teamwork with social workers.

The social worker's role can be classified into three parts:

(a) A statutory responsibility based on Acts of Parliament, especially in relation to child care and mental health. The statutory work of the social worker in mental health is described in some sections of the Mental Health Act, e.g. Sections 25, 26 and 29.

(b) Social Services Departments have access to numerous resources, such as grants towards telephone installation and towards adapting houses to meet the needs of the chronically handicapped in the community. They have responsibilities placed on them by the 1970 Disabled Persons Act. In addition, social workers are often able to put patients (whom they call clients) in touch with numerous voluntary organisations or bodies who may be able to provide advice, resources, or support.

(c) The most important of the professional skills of social workers is called 'case work'. This requires an analysis of the client's/patient's

personality, his relationship to his family and contacts and particularly
the relationship with the professional worker, and then using these to
help the client develop insight and the ability to cope with his life. To
do this social workers use a counselling relationship with clients, often
of a non-directive type.

The essence of counselling is that the individual is offered the
opportunity to talk about his problems. The aim is to help the person to
help himself. The relationship is non-authoritarian in the sense that it
is not intended that the professional should give the client or patient
orders, but should be available for long periods of time to share the
problems of the client, to listen sympathetically, to probe, challenge
and to question, and to work with the client in a sense of partnership
to achieve a shared solution to the problems. Advice and access to outside resources is part of the counsellor's contribution, but the whole
exercise is designed primarily to promote the autonomy of the
individual.

In the past this approach has been distinctive of social workers and
represented one of the greatest contributions to the caring professions.
Both doctors and nurses have tended to operate on a strictly authoritarian model, although many general practitioners have for years
eschewed the notion of 'doctors' orders' and have advocated 'talking
with patients and deciding together' (Batten, 1961).

Nowadays general practice, especially through vocational training
and its own developing literature, is drawing on the approach of social
work. More and more general practitioners are seeking to adopt the
counselling method in their own consultations. There is now a new
society to promote counselling in medicine. The address is 4 Greenland
Road, London NW1.

Paine (1976) has described how a group of part-time social workers
can function effectively as a social-work team in association with one
practice. Numerous other developments are occurring in different parts
of the country. The literature on co-operation and collaboration is
increasing rapidly (Brook & Temperley, 1976; Graham & Sher, 1976;
and several contributions by Ratoff *et al*., 1974).

6. Remedial Therapists

Remedial therapists are only rarely members of the general practice
team but signs of their inclusion are appearing. Freedman *et al*. (1975),
Waters *et al*. (1975), have described working with physiotherapists in
general practice and two of us have links with remedial therapists in

general practice. Certainly the traditions and skills of these paramedicals seem ideally suited to co-operation and we recommend that opportunities should be sought and taken where available to promote collaboration.

The remedialists can offer an advisory service on rehabilitation, including that for handicapped children, for patients with strokes and for those with disabling disease. The kind of physiotherapy services in the practice described in the two papers recommended above include the mobilisation and rehabilitation of patients in their own homes.

Remedial therapy may emerge as a new combined profession incorporating the separate skills of physiotherapy, occupational therapy and speech therapy. If the benefits of systematic relaxation therapy are confirmed as a treatment for both physical and emotional conditions, remedial therapists could further extend their role. Patel (1976) has reported lowering blood pressure and blood fats by relaxation exercises.

Appointment of Attached Staff

We believe that the relationship between doctors and nurses is so close that it is highly desirable that general practitioners should always attend the selection committees when attached staff are being appointed to work in their practices. Many if not most of the progressive health authorities are already offering this and we believe that it is important that general practices should ensure that these invitations are always accepted and that at least one partner attends to represent the practice. Our experience in Devon has been most encouraging and the offer to attend selection committees has been much appreciated.

Relationships within the team need to be analysed carefully. It is generally agreed that good teamwork may take years to develop—hence the importance of ensuring that attachments of health visitors and district nurses should be long-term and not altered unless absolutely necessary. We believe that it is to the advantage of the attached staff if they have a well-equipped and pleasantly furnished room of their own, a secure place and base in the practice itself.

The pattern of the future of general practice in Britain is already clear and it is now virtually certain that general practitioners will work in ever-closer association with colleagues in other caring professions. The sooner we get to know the skills and assets of the other professions the better. We need to analyse, understand and promote good teamwork for the years ahead.

The Future

Teamwork in general practice has come to stay. Even the solo practitioner now usually has one or more secretaries, a receptionist and often a dispenser. He or she will usually have regular meetings with an attached district nurse, health visitor, midwife and, increasingly, a social worker. Both the number and proportion of single-handed general practitioners in Britain has been steadily declining for many years. The proportion of practitioners in group practice is growing and the proportion in partnerships of five or more is rising sharply (DHSS, 1977).

We therefore believe that most trainees can expect to work in partnership and to become members of general-practice teams.

Groups and practices develop over the years a group identity or personality of their own. There are happy and hectic teams, complaining teams and aggressive or miserable teams. The kind of team identity which emerges depends on the individuals involved, but the general practitioners will always have a special responsibility for leadership. Good team leaders are usually made, not born. That is why teamwork needs study, so that its principles can be identified and learnt. Group behaviour is increasingly being studied in vocational training courses and trainers' workshops.

References and Further Reading

Balint, M. *The Doctor, His Patient and the Illness*, 2nd edition (London: Pitman, 1964).

Batten, L. James Mackenzie Lecture 1960. *Journal of the College of General Practitioners*, 4 (1961), pp. 5-18.

Bolden, K.J. & Morgan, D.C. 'Moving to a health centre – the effect on workload and patients', *Journal of the Royal College of General Practitioners*, 25 (1975), pp. 527-31.

Brook, A. & Temperley, J. 'Psychotherapist attached to general practice', *Journal of the Royal College of General Practitioners*, 26 (1976), pp. 86-94.

Department of Health and Social Security. *Health and Social Services Statistics for England for 1977* (London: HMSO, 1977).

Forman, J.A.S. & Fairbairn, E. *Social Casework in General Practice* (London: OUP, 1968).

Freedman, O.P. *et al.* 'Physiotherapy in general practice', *Journal of the Royal College of General Practitioners*, 25 (1975), pp. 587-91.

Goldberg, E.M. & Neil, J.E. *Social Work in General Practice* (London: Allen & Unwin, 1972).

Graham, H. & Sher, M. 'Social work and general practice', *Journal of the Royal College of General Practitioners*, 26 (1976), pp. 95-105.

Gray, D.J. Pereira. James Mackenzie Lecture 1977. 'Feeling at home', *Journal of the Royal College of General Practitioners*, 28 (1978), pp. 6-17.

Harris, E. & Jones, R.V.H. 'District nurses. How many in AD 2000?' *Nursing Mirror*, 2 (1977), pp. 35-6.

Hart, C.R. (ed.). *Child Care in General Practice* (Edinburgh: E. & S. Livingstone, 1977).

Lamberts, H. & Riphagen, F.F. 'The team in primary health care', *Journal of the Royal College of General Practitioners*, 25 (1975), pp. 745-52.

Paine, T.F. 'Social workers in general practice', *Journal of the Royal College of General Practitioners*, 26 (1976), pp. 695-7.

Patel, C.H. 'Behaviour modification therapy', *Journal of the Royal College of General Practitioners*, 26 (1976), pp. 211-15.

Ratoff, L., Rose, A. & Smith, C. 'Social workers and general practitioners', *Journal of the Royal College of General Practitioners*, 24 (1974), pp. 750-60.

Waters, W.H.R., Sanderman, J.M. & Lunn, J.E. 'A four-year prospective study of the work of the practice nurse in the treatment-room of a South Yorkshire practice', *British Medical Journal*, 280 (1980), pp. 87-9.

Waters, W.H.R., Udy, S.C. & Lunn, J.E. 'Organising a Physiotherapy service in general practice', *Journal of the Royal College of General Practitioners*, 25 (1975), pp. 576-84.

7 THE PRINCIPLES OF MANAGEMENT IN THE PRACTICE

> The essential unit of medical practice is the occasion when, in the intimacy of the consulting room or sick room, a person who is ill or believes himself to be ill, seeks the advice of a doctor whom he trusts. This is the consultation and all else in the practice of medicine derives from it (Spence, 1960).

The consultation as defined above has always remained the focus of general practice and the purpose of practice organisation or management is to promote the quality of that consultation so that the maximum benefit is obtained by the patient. This statement of practice management sounds simple, but if this primary aim is not constantly remembered there is always a danger that organisation and management will become an end in itself and develop into a self-perpetuating and increasingly expensive machine.

In Chapters 2 and 11 we stress the fact that general practitioners are independent contractors and are self-employed. We are, therefore, responsible for the organisation of our own partnership or firm equivalent of directors of businesses.

Medical practice is one of the few situations in our society where major decisions about people's lives are taken regularly. Eimerl & Pearson (1976) have shown that the speed of decision-taking in modern general practice is probably as quick as in any other profession.

Business management is now an established discipline and it is necessary for practitioners as responsible partners to understand the principles of good organisation. Organisation management, therefore, should form part of the training of all future general practitioners.

General Principles

There are several general principles which can be applied to all systems of organisation and management in all general practices:

(1) The decision-making process should be clear and understood.
(2) Appointment of staff should not be made in a haphazard fashion

77

without unanimous agreement among partners.

(3) Practice rules should be absolutely clear to all members of the staff and the reasons for the rules understood.

(4) The organisation should promote individual initiative and experiment by all members of staff.

(5) There should be personal contact between those in authority (the general-practitioner partners) and those who are employed by them.

(6) Delegation should be planned individually in the light of the particular skills of each member of staff.

(7) Meetings should be held frequently enough to prevent difficulties becoming grievances.

(8) Management should initiate and encourage feedback on the working of all practice systems.

(9) Information should be shared.

1. Clarifying the Decision-making Process

By definition the final point of the decision-making process in general practice in Britain is the partnership meeting. Both in law as the employers, and as individuals 'collectively and severally responsible' to the Inland Revenue Authorities, the partners in a group practice are legally and financially responsible for the practice. The partnership meeting is where the buck stops. In law all partners are liable for the sins and omissions of all partners; patients can sue the whole partnership if they choose. This means that the partnership meetings, their organ-isation, their frequency, their minutes, and the way their decisions are translated into action are crucial in every group practice. The frequency of meetings must be by agreement between partners but normally they should not be less than monthly and arrangements have to be flexible enough for extra meetings to deal with particular problems. The arrangement for partnership meetings is often specified in partnership agreements.

Decisions taken at partnership meetings must be recorded in writing. We find one of the most effective methods is to indicate after each discussion the initials of the partner responsible, e.g. 'It was agreed to explore costs of buying an ECG machine. Action X.' The list of 'actions' forms the 'matters arising' for the agenda of the next meeting. There are several reasons why written records are necessary for partnership meetings:

(1) These are business meetings, at which as shown throughout this book decisions about people (staff) and substantial sums of money are taken. Most partnerships of three partners in Britain have an annual turnover of about £60,000 and bigger groups can easily exceed £100,000 turnover each year. Throughout the world it is good business practice to keep a written record of business meetings and the decisions taken by executives.

(2) Human nature being what it is, decisions tend to get left – often just by inertia. It is usually easier to do nothing rather than something and this may mean that new ideas and policies get perpetually postponed. Older doctors especially tend to defer changes; a decision to postpone is still a decision!

By simply having a written agenda at least each month and by listing as items on the agenda all the decisions reached at the previous meeting, an automatic tightening up of procedure is achieved relatively painlessly. This can be particularly important for new young principals, particularly vocational trainees, who on entering a practice often bring many new and stimulating ideas. It is remarkable how much gets done a few days *before* partnership meetings!

(3) If decisions are not minuted in writing some will be forgotten.

(4) Written minutes remind all the partners that they are working as business partners and will make what is implicit explicit. It will soon become apparent if one partner is being left with all the responsibility.

Partnerships in which there are no written minutes often function with one dominant partner who runs the practice. The 'Managing Director' model may work well for a few years but eventually will lead to the other partner or partners becoming either resentful, dependent, or isolated, all of which we regard as unsatisfactory. New partners need to establish what exactly is partnership business, and what decisions can be delegated to different members of the staff. In time, however, the policy should be clarified not only in the minds of all the partners but also in the minds of all the staff, in terms of the kind of decision to be taken by the partners: policy decisions about appointing partners or staff; policy about clinical management of patients or about organisations or individuals outside the practice; policy on accepting new patients; policy in relation to financial shares, and about financial management, depreciation and expenditure on equipment, maintenance and repairs.

We have mentioned earlier and will discuss again in Chapter 11 the importance of the partnership agreement which controls the broad legal framework within which the practice partnership exists, but regular

monthly meetings and above all day-to-day contact between partners
build up the human relationships which determine how any group of
partners functions as a team. The management principle, however, is
that the staff should have a general idea of where the buck stops, how
the practice is organised and where and why the main decisions are taken.

Difficulties in Decision-making

One of the most important variables affecting decision-making is the
number of people involved. Given the desirability of informing, discussing
and always consulting those affected by decisions, the advantage of keeping groups small becomes clear. The complications of achieving decisions,
without imposing them through a hierarchy of authority, rise geomet-
rically with the number of people. Small is beautiful!

Delays

Similarly, one of the worst aspects of management in big organisations
is the delay which so often takes place before an answer, any answer,
appears. A good decision may become only a moderate, if not a bad
decision, if it is long delayed. Partners should always be conscious of
how long it takes for a decision to be acted upon in the practice.

2. Appointing Staff

Appointing members of staff is always important. Everyone in the
premises has access to notes and confidential information and in a small
group of people working together the personality and the behaviour
of one member of a team always affects the others. A chain is no
stronger than its weakest link, so the partners must vet every single
link in the chain of the team.

  We recommend that all partners should normally attend all interviews
and should be joined by the practice manager or senior member of staff
who will have to work closely with the new person. It is useful to have
in the practice a typed list of standard questions to clarify at interview.
One such check list is in Appendix D.

3. Rules and their Reasons

All families and groups of people need to have their own rules and the
bigger the group and the more complicated its task the greater is the
need for some set of rules. The general principle of management for
general-practitioner partners, however, is quite simple — rules should be
as few as possible so that staff are restricted as little as possible. A rule
should be introduced only when it is a necessary safeguard to patients.

Whenever a rule is introduced, it should always be fully discussed with whoever is involved; above all there is an obligation on those in authority, i.e. the partners, to explain fully and repeatedly the reasons for it. Finally, all important rules should be recorded in writing and should be available to staff who have to operate them.

For example, many practitioners have found that occasionally messages from patients are forgotten unless rules are enforced. It is common in practices to have a rule that all requests for home visits are recorded in writing in a suitable book and the time of the call noted. If part-time staff are changing over during the day the exact time of responsibility should be mutually agreed and kept on the notice board.

4. Encouraging Staff Initiative

The employer—employee relationship is a great responsibility for the employer. General practitioners are fortunate working in relatively small and enclosed systems. We do not have to face the great problems of authority and hierarchy which occur in other parts of the Health Service and in many other organisations.

It is a useful principle in general practice to avoid a hierarchy of more than three ranks. The organisation of partner/senior secretary/receptionist/ or junior secretary is probably as much as is comfortable or necessary. General practice is built up on individual relationships between doctor and patient and this should be the model for organisation as well. Organisation often works best with a single practitioner with a single secretary, but obviously modifications are necessary in big groups.

The doctors must seek to encourage initiative. Ideas and criticisms should always be encouraged, carefully considered, and if possible, implemented. If a member of staff proposes a different way of doing something and the partners are uncertain whether the new method offers any real advantage, there is much to be said for allowing the experiment. It will provide a healthy challenge to the inherent conservatism of the practice and will inevitably involve the member of staff actively in the organisation. It will promote interest in the experiment among other members of the staff, which is all to the good. Organisations where the staff never make any suggestions or where such suggestions are never implemented will soon lose the better members of the staff or at least lose their enthusiasm and interest.

Just as the model of the relationship between general practitioner and patient strives towards equality and partnership, so the general-practitioner partner as an employer should strive for a partnership relationship with his staff.

5. Personal Contact

Most human beings in most organisations make regular contact with other people. Most of the doctors who work in general practice and most of their staff do their job because they like working with people. Strangely enough, however, the high turnover of patients and the pressures of general practice stress the administrative systems of management to the point that the members of the team may sometimes have little or no time to talk to each other and may find themselves rushing home after evening surgery exchanging only a few words.

In particular, doctors cannot allow the stresses and strains of life to be dealt with by 'taking it out' on whoever happens to be present at the time. Such behaviour by doctors only creates guilt and anger in the staff who in turn may 'take it out' on patients.

It is a general principle of management that a good employer sees his staff as individuals with their particular strengths and weaknesses and gets to know them as individual human beings. There is no substitute for personal contact, such as having time occasionally for a chat or staying to have a cup of coffee when the surgery has finished. If we wish our staff to provide a personal service for patients, we owe it to them to care for them ourselves. As a general rule each member of staff should be entitled to a fixed time in the week to discuss any problems with the partner concerned.

6. Delegation

Specialisation of labour is a fundamental principle of modern organisation and the division of labour is one of the principal devices for improving output in organisations. Obvious examples include typing and filing, where it is almost certainly true that most professional secretaries type letters better than most doctors!

Allied to this principle is the theory of delegation. If there is work that can be equally well done by a non-doctor, then it is more efficient for it to be done by a less highly trained person, e.g. filing clerks file the letters, which is more efficient than the doctor doing it himself. This principle holds true as long as the doctor's training is longer than that of the filing clerk and as long as the doctors are more highly paid.

The principle of delegation should not just be thought of in terms of organisation but is equally applicable to clinical work. *The Practice Nurse* published by the Royal College of General Practitioners (*Reports from General Practice*, No. 10) suggested the possible clinical scope of the practice nurse as long as ten years ago.

Delegation, or who does what in a practice team, is discussed in

Chapter 6. However, the management principle is that it should be flexible, dynamic, and subject to constant review because the history of medicine shows that what is considered to be a task appropriate for a doctor at one time is often equally generally recognised to be the nurse's work at another.

7. Regular Meetings

In addition to individual personal contact, it is a general principle of management that meetings should be held often enough to allow members of the staff of any organisation to express their ideas and feelings in the context of a group with their seniors or employers. In the short hierarchy that is characteristic of general-practice organisation, this means meetings between the partners and the staff. There is no general rule about how often these ought to take place but there are two guiding principles: the staff themselves should choose the frequency and the doctors should fit in with them. The appearance of numerous complaints and grievances usually represents a symptom of inadequate communication and a sign that meetings are too infrequent.

In one of our practices the staff meet the partners once a quarter and the different groups within the practice team, such as the three part-time SRNs, meet the partners about every two months. In addition, there are short fixed weekly meetings of the health visitor, district nurses and the practice manager, in order to deal with day-to-day decisions.

8. Feedback

It is useful to consider practice organisation in terms of system analysis. Practices are living growing groups, capable of developing or regressing. One of the most important management principles is that those who are responsible for decision-making at all levels should be regularly supplied with information about the consequences of their previous decisions. Feedback of factual information about, for example, the list sizes and prescription costs are routine through the NHS in all practices. These rough and ready data supplied to general practitioners through the National Health Service are seriously inadequate as a basis for practice.

Modern general practitioners expect much more detailed and much more regular feedback to partners than this and it is the responsibility of partners themselves to organise systems so that this information is regularly generated as part of the routine day-to-day work of the practice and is not regarded by the staff who do it as an unnecessary and additional chore.

What kind of information is useful? First and foremost the size of the
list and the way that it is changing, the total number of patients and the
frequency with which they consult, is almost basic information if any
rational attempt is to be made to organise an appointment system.
Keeping regular accounts of all consultations and visits is the only way
to detect developing trends and to compare the practice with the results
published by others.

We will describe some simple systems of financial analysis in Chapters
9 and 10. The relevant principle here, however, is that only by feeding
back information about what is happening and what are the consequences,
is it possible to discuss, adapt and improve the financial system. Partners
today are entitled to expect regular returns on all the main activities in
their practice – not just for themselves, but for all the partners. Similarly,
members of staff who run parts of the practice should be supplied with
feedback about the results.

9. Sharing Information

Teamwork is discussed in Chapter 6. However, it is already clear that the
majority of general practitioners in the United Kingdom in the future are
going to work in groups with what is likely to be an increasing number
of secretaries, nurses, receptionists, and health visitors.

Communication can be defined as sharing information and making
decisions. Most of this chapter so far has been concerned primarily with
decision-making. Sharing information is, however, equally important.
Failure to share information is probably the greatest weakness in
general practice organisation in Britain today.

The problem arises because although the general-practitioner partners
automatically discuss between themselves all the important organisational
issues by virtue of their partnership, and although the senior practice
secretary or practice manager is likely to know most of the news by
virtue of her job, there is nevertheless a tendency for other members of
the team to be left out. Information is not always shared automatically
and one of the tests of a good organisation is to assess the formal ways
it may have for sharing information among all those who work in the
practice.

Behaviour of the staff can be a symptom of failure. 'Oh, I didn't
know that,' particularly if repeated, or worse still, 'Nobody ever tells
me anything' are comments that give a clear indication to the general-
practitioner partners that counter-action is needed and more organised
methods must be introduced for sharing information.

Most important is the direct and personal discussion between partners and different members of the team. There is, as has been shown above, no substitute for this. It should be the responsibility moreover of all the partners to do it. However, there is much routine information which tends to be forgotten in such discussion or which may not be directly relevant until later. Responsibility may be allocated to a senior member of the staff, preferably the practice organiser, administrator, or senior secretary, and she should have as part of her work the responsibility of ensuring that other members of the staff are informed of important information which is relevant to the working of the practice.

The practice meetings described above also serve as an opportunity for information to be shared and questions to be asked by all members of the staff. In the context of information-sharing, staff notice-boards are also helpful. In one of our practices we list the workload figures and the changes in frequency of home visits and consultations which are all prepared by one member of the staff, the records clerk, and presented periodically to the partners. By putting the annual returns on the notice-board for all members of the staff to see, everybody shares the information generated. Sharing information does not just happen automatically; it is part of the responsibility of management to plan for this to happen regularly.

Changing Systems

The principles of management outlined in this chapter are accepted by all the four authors of this book, and govern the working of our practices. There are, however, many general practices where some or all of these principles are neither accepted nor operated.

We do not believe that management systems, however desirable, can be imposed suddenly. On the whole, general practice has always progressed best by evolution rather than revolution and changes in organisation, however good, are usually best introduced slowly with a great deal of discussion with all the people concerned.

Doctor–Staff Relationships

General practice has already made a huge contribution to medicine by emphasising the tremendous importance of the doctor–patient relationship (Balint, 1964, Browne & Freeling, 1976). General practitioners have shown that this relationship or interaction not only affects the way patients and doctors feel but directly influences the quality of care the patient receives.

The principles of managing staff are directly analogous to the principles of managing patients and each of the sections discussed above has a parallel in the doctor—patient relationship. In summary, it all boils down to liking and trusting staff and treating them as we would like to be treated ourselves.

References

Balint, M. *The Doctor, His Patient and the Illness*, 2nd edition (London: Pitman, 1964).
Browne, K. & Freeling, P. *The Doctor-Patient Relationship*, 2nd edition (London: Longman, 1976).
Eimerl, T. & Pearson, R.J.C. *British Medical Journal*, 2 (1976), pp. 1549-54.
Royal College of General Practitioners. *The Practice Nurse. Reports from General Practice*, No. 10 (London: Royal College of General Practitioners, 1970).
Spence, J. in *The Purpose and Practice of Medicine* (London: OUP, 1960).

PART FOUR: MONEY

8 FINANCE: MONEY IN

It is only comparatively recently, since family doctors began to organise themselves into larger groups and partnerships, that the importance of having clear and accurate financial accounts has been generally appreciated. Larger practices result in more complex organisation, higher shared income and higher shared expenses. It is important for the partnership that each partner should have a clear idea of where the money comes from and where the money goes. In this chapter possible sources of practice income are discussed. In Chapter 9 the subject of practice expenses is considered.

General practitioners have three types of income:

(1) Personal income from sources other than medical practice.
(2) Private income from medical work outside the National Health Service.
(3) Income from the National Health Service.

The 'practice income' of a general practitioner, whether he is in partnership or in single-handed practice, consists of income from the medical work undertaken in 'practice time'.

1. Personal Income

This is unconnected with the practice and does not usually involve partners. For most such income (e.g. interest from stocks or shares owned personally by the general practitioner) poses no problem of definition. There may be, however, some difficulty in deciding whether income from such activities as writing or lecturing is 'personal' or has taken place in 'practice time' and should therefore be classed as practice income. This is a matter which should be covered in the partnership agreement.

2a. Private Income for Most General Practitioners

1. Insurance Examinations and Reports

Medical reports are used by insurance companies to assess the risk (and therefore the premium) for life and sickness insurance policies. These reports may either be full reports involving examination of the patient, or short reports on the medical history of the patient culled from the practitioner's knowledge and the medical record. For some general practitioners who are medical examiners for large insurance companies, these examinations may form a considerable proportion of their work. Nevertheless, most general practitioners do some insurance work.

Satisfactory medical reports are also required by insurance companies before they will insure an elderly person to drive a car. Companies vary regarding the age at which they start demanding a medical examination, and the frequency with which this has to be repeated. It is usual for an elderly driver to go to his own general practitioner for this examination but it is quite in order for him to go to any doctor of his choice.

2. Other Medical Examinations and Certificates

Medical examinations are required or requested for many other purposes, e.g. when applying for a heavy goods vehicle driving licence, for fitness to take up a job, or to go on a diving course. For all certificates involving a medical examination which are not covered by National Insurance Regulations (F Med 3), the general practitioner is entitled to payment.

Although vaccination and immunisation are procedures to which a patient is entitled under the Health Service, the provision of a certificate stating that these procedures have been carried out also attracts a fee.

3. Legal Reports

Most general practitioners will appear in Court as a witness at some time in their professional lives, probably as a witness of fact rather than an expert witness. They will also be required on occasions to give evidence at a Coroner's Court. For these attendances they are entitled to a fee.

In common with any other citizen who may have been involved in such episodes as an assault, car accidents, or drunken brawls, a general practitioner may be asked by the police to provide a report as a witness. For such a report the practitioner is not entitled to a fee. But should a report be requested by the police which involves expression of a medical opinion then a fee should be charged. Reports made at the request of the police after a doctor has examined someone at a police station fall

into this category. In most cities and larger towns these examinations
are carried out by the 'police surgeon' (who is usually a local general
practitioner), but in country districts there may be no such appointment. If a person who is detained in a police station asks to see his
own general practitioner, then that consultation and examination does
not fall under the normal terms of service and the practitioner is
entitled to a fee.

Solicitors may also ask for reports, usually about a patient who is
involved in litigation. The fee for this type of report is not standard,
but depends upon the complexity of the report and the amount of
time the practitioner has to spend on it. As these rates tend to vary,
advice concerning the current rate can usually be obtained from the
local branch of the Law Society.

4. Cremation Fees

The Brodrick Report, published in 1971, suggested major changes in the
procedure to be followed before a body could be cremated. At present,
however, the cremation certificate consists of two parts: the first part
is signed by the doctor who attended the deceased during their last
illness; the second part is signed by an independent practitioner, who
cannot be a partner of the doctor who signed the first part and who must
have been fully registered for five years. For each part a fee is paid by
the executors of the deceased. Usually the undertaker settles this with
the doctor on their behalf.

For many of the services referred to above the scale of fees is standard
and agreed. The British Medical Association publish a booklet called
Fees for Part-time Medical Services which is regularly updated. In many
practices, however, the scale of fees suggested by the BMA may not be
used—some doctors charging patients less than the agreed rate. If this
is so, then great care should be taken to write on the notes *exactly* how
much has been charged for which service and when, otherwise misunderstandings ensue between patient and doctor and between one partner
and another.

2b. Private Income for Some General Practitioners

Many of the medical activities in which general practitioners indulge
attract no fee at all. Examples are the life-boat service, acting as medical
officer at various sporting functions, or as adviser to the Red Cross or
St John's Ambulance. But in most practices at least one principal has an

outside appointment of some sort. These appointments vary enormously in the responsibilities involved, in the time taken, and in the income received. There are certain broad categories of such appointments and sources of 'private' income.

1. Appointments with Local Authorities

These may be sessional appointments in the medical department for such activities as developmental clinics, or may be appointments to other local authority departments, such as the police or fire brigade.

2. Medical Officers to Schools

Many different types of school have part-time officers who are usually general practitioners. These include boarding-schools, special schools for the handicapped and approved schools. The duties involve not only medical care of individual pupils but also advice to the school authorities on such things as diet, hygiene, and all matters concerning 'public health' in the school setting. Chapter 14 includes further discussion on this subject.

3. Industrial Medical Officers

Large firms employ medical officers as full-time employees, but many medium-sized or small firms employ local general practitioners as part-time advisers. They may be responsible for advising the employer on a prospective employee's fitness for work, on industrial health risks, on general health education matters, and on such matters as the early retirement of employees on grounds of ill-health.

4. Hospital Appointments

Many general practitioners are employed in the hospital service on a sessional basis. Before 1976 the appointment was as a clinical assistant but since that date appointments have also been made to the hospital practitioner grade. Hospital practitioner grade appointments are permanent, but for a job to be so recognised it has to fulfil certain criteria of function and responsibility. The doctor applying for such a post has also to meet certain criteria.

There has been considerable confusion within the profession since this grade was negotiated by the GMSC for general practitioners—and this confusion has not so far (1980) been fully resolved. Until the situation is clarified it is particularly important that a general practitioner applying for a part-time hospital appointment should enquire fully into the terms and circumstances of that appointment.

5. Appointments to Other Bodies

Large organisations, such as the Post Office, the IBA, and the BBC, have local part-time medical officers who are usually general practitioners.

6. Teaching and Lecturing

Over the past decade there has been a steady increase in the numbers of general practitioners involved in lecturing and teaching. To the staple diet of lectures to the Red Cross or St John's Ambulance Brigade are now added lectures at postgraduate centres, to medical societies, and to meetings of paramedical workers. There is a growing realisation, both by general practitioners themselves and by other health workers, that general practitioners have unrivalled experience in diagnosis and management at that interface where a person becomes a patient. Although it is probably true to say that few general practitioners find lecturing easy, it is inevitable that the demand for articulate general practitioner lecturers will grow.

7. Private Patients

Before 1948 most general practitioners obtained a sizeable proportion of their income from private patients. There were many who had no 'panel patients' and obtained all their income this way. The position is now reversed. There are many practices which do not accept private patients. For those that do, it is usually accepted that the commodity which the private patient buys is convenience rather than quality of medical care. Each general practitioner who does accept private patients should keep a day book. In this the service and the fee to be charged are noted under the appropriate date, so that accounts can be sent out at regular (usually quarterly) intervals.

In some partnerships the proportion of time spent in the practice and the proportion spent on outside appointments varies widely from partner to partner. It is essential for harmony within a partnership that the arrangements for the distribution of this 'private income' are clearly understood from the beginning. It is also essential that when consideration is being given to one partner taking on an additional commitment outside the practice that the implications for all partners are fully discussed and understood.

3. Income from the National Health Service

For the majority of general practitioners, private and personal income is a minor part of the total income. The largest part of most general practitioners' income comes from work done within the Health Service.

As a principal in general practice a doctor is paid by his Family Practitioner Committee under five main headings. In the following section the relevant paragraph number of the Red Book (the name of which is strictly *The Statement of Fees and Allowances payable to General Practitioners in England and Wales*) is placed after each category of payment so that reference can be made if more information is needed. The fees and allowances for the current year can also be found in paras 1 and 1/Sch. 1 of the Red Book (see Chapter 15 for further details of this).

1. Fixed Sum. Paid to each Principal in Practice

(a) Basic Allowance (12.1). This is paid to each principal with more than 1,000 patients on his list. A proportion of the allowance is paid to those with less than 1,000 patients. The justification for this payment is that it is to cover the 'expenses of having a practice' but the various expenses have never been specifically named or itemised. It is fair to say that some members of the profession, both in general practice and in the DHSS, regard this as part-salary.

(b) Supplementary Practice Allowance (22.1). This is an extension of the basic practice allowance. It is paid to each general practitioner with more than 1,000 patients on his list who provides an 'out of hours' service (viz. night and weekend cover).

2. Fees Based on Number of Patients

(a) Capitation Fee (21.1). A fee is paid for each patient on the general practitioner's list aged 64 years and under. A slightly higher fee is paid for those aged 65-74, and a higher fee again for those aged over 75.

(b) Supplementary Capitation Fee (23.1). Payment is made to cover the extra work done by a general practitioner for the patients on his list outside 'normal working hours'. There is a capitation payment for the number of patients on his list over 1,000. This is distinct from the night visit fee which is an item-of-service payment.

(c) Temporary Resident's Fee (32.1). This is a fee paid for treating visitors who are in the district for more than 24 hours but less than three months. The rate is lower for a patient who stays less than a fortnight than for one who stays longer. There is a form FP19/EC19

on which this fee is claimed for each temporary resident.

(d) Contraceptive Fee (29.1). This is a fee paid for those patients who sign on for contraceptive services. At present the patient has to sign an annual application for these services (FP1001), which is sent to the Family Practitioner Committee after being countersigned by the doctor to indicate that he has agreed to accept the patient on his contraceptive list. There is a higher rate for fitting an IUD than for general services.

3. Item of Service

Item-of-service fees are paid to the general practitioner for work he does in addition to the general medical care for patients on his list. They are a motley collection; some are paid for preventive measures, such as immunisation, which are blessed by the DHSS (and thereafter called 'public policy'). Others are paid to general practitioners when they perform certain specific (usually unpleasant) duties. Current payments are made for the following services:

(a)   vaccination and immunisation (27.1)
(b)   cervical cytology (28.1)
(c)   night visit fee (24.1)
(d)   maternity services and miscarriage (31.1)
(e)   arrest of dental haemorrhage (35.1)
(f)   emergency treatment fee (33.1)
(g)   anaesthetic fee (34.1)

4. Fees Based on a Practitioner's Qualifications

These fees are dependent on either the age, experience, and training of the individual general practitioner, or on his appointment as a general practitioner trainer.

The fees paid for age, experience and training are paid automatically to all who fulfil the criteria. The would-be trainer, however, has to apply to the local Regional Adviser for General Practice for recognition before he is accepted as a trainer. He then has to undergo a selection procedure agreed by the Joint Committee on Postgraduate Training for General Practice. The fees for training are paid to him only for the periods during which he has a trainee.

The references to the fees which are based on practitioners' qualifications are as follows:

(a)   vocational training allowance (17.1)

    (b)   seniority allowance (16.1)
    (c)   postgraduate training allowance (37.1)
    (d)   trainer allowance (38.1)

5. Fees for Type or Position of Practice

Practices in different parts of the British Isles may attract payments depending on their location. The additional expense involved for the general practitioner who has a geographically large practice is recognised in rural practice payments.

(a) Rural Practice Payments (43.1). Payments are made to practitioners from a special fund for all those patients who live three miles or more from the main surgery. Most of these payments are made to rural or semi-rural practitioners but those doctors who practise in urban areas may also claim payment if the criteria of the Red Book are met.

Patients attract so many 'units' depending on the distance they live from the main surgery and difficulty of access. Grounds for claiming difficulty of access include narrow roads liable to frequent obstruction (by, for example, livestock, farm vehicles or floods) or the fact that the house cannot be reached by car so that the practitioner can claim 'walking units'. Special arrangements exist for particularly isolated patients, such as those living on small islands.

In all these circumstances it is the doctor who is responsible for claiming the appropriate units from the Family Practitioner Committee. Clearly considerable income may be lost if he does not claim those units to which he is entitled.

(b) Dispensing Fees (44.1). Dispensing doctors can choose to be paid either by a capitation or by a drug tariff system. The majority of practitioners choose the latter. Practitioners who do not normally dispense can claim payment for certain injections and vaccines which they administer personally to patients (44.13). Dispensing practice is discussed further in Appendix F.

(c) Designated Area Allowance (14.1). There are two types of designated area allowance. For type I the area must have been designated for at least three years. For type II, as well as having been designated for at least one year, the average list size in the area must be 3,000 patients or more. Type II attracts a higher allowance.

(d) Initial Practice Allowance (40.1). There are four different types of

initial practice allowance labelled A, B, C and D. They are paid to
doctors who set up practice in designated areas or in areas where it is
agreed by the DHSS and the Medical Practices Committee that a large
increase in population may be expected within a few years (such as large
housing developments or new towns).

(e) Inducement Allowance (45.1). This is paid as an inducement to
maintain a practice in a sparsely populated area, such as the highlands
of Scotland.

(f) Group Practice Allowance (15.1). Three or more doctors practising
in association (but not necessarily in partnership) may be eligible for
a group practice allowance provided the criteria laid down in the Red
Book are met.

6. Reimbursements

In addition to these direct payments, general practitioners are reimbursed
for the rent they pay for their premises, whether these are rents for
health centre premises (53.1), privately rented premises, or notional
rents for premises which the general practitioners own (51.1). The
District Valuer has to inspect the premises and agree an appropriate
rent before this reimbursement is made.

Repayment is also made for a proportion (currently 70 per cent) of
the salary paid to members of the ancillary staff employed by general
practitioners, provided that certain conditions are met (52.1), for
National Insurance contributions in respect of employed staff (52.8) and
for certain staff pension contributions (52.8 and 52.9).

The Family Practitioner Committee normally makes payments to
general practitioners quarterly in arrears. Any practice can, however,
apply to have a proportion of their expected payment made in advance.
Many practices have arranged for payment to be made at the end of
the first and second months of each quarter, with the balance paid at
the end of the quarter. As expenses are incurred and have to be paid
throughout the quarter this arrangement has the great advantage of
providing cash nearer to the time that the service is provided and the
expense incurred.

Average Income

To give some idea of the proportion of income that the 'average'
general practitioner earns under each heading, an analysis of the
'average general practitioner's income' for 1975/6 based on figures
provided by the DHSS) is provided in Appendix E. It is interesting to
note that for 1975/6 the proportion of income as a national average
under the headings used earlier was:

Fixed sum:	21%
Capitation:	45%
Item of service:	6%
GP qualifications:	6%
Type or position of practice:	12%

The remaining 10 per cent was made up by reimbursements and
minor items.

The interest of this information for the individual practitioner is
that it can be both enlightening and profitable to compare the figures
for his practice with the national average. For those areas in which he
is below the average it may be possible to increase his income with a
little planning. There is further discussion of this point in Chapters 10
and 13.

Summing Up

All this may appear very complicated to the new entrant into general
practice. These arrangements have been evolved over the years. Each
paragraph in the Red Book represents months of negotiation between
the profession and the DHSS. There is no doubt, however, that because
of a combination of ignorance and idleness, many general practitioners
have in the past not received the fees which they have earned.

There are certainly some general practitioners who have not claimed
reimbursement of the rent of branch surgeries. There are others who
have claimed a temporary resident fee when a larger emergency treatment fee was appropriate. Medical men, and in particular general
practitioners, are notoriously careless when it comes to running the
business side of their practices. Because so many of us are not
temperamentally inclined to 'chase the pennies', one solution is to
delegate a senior member of the ancillary staff to scrutinise the amendments to the Red Book (called SFA followed by a number) as they
arrive and make sure that the partners are aware of their significance.

Another method may be for each partner to take it in turns to be responsible for this.

Whatever method is adopted it is important that practitioners are aware of the significance of the Red Book and its amendments in view of the direct effect that changes have on their practice income.

9   FINANCE: MONEY OUT

'That's the way the money goes;
Pop goes the weasel.'

The expenses involved in running a practice are of two kinds: running
expenses and capital expenses. Capital expenses are defined by accountants as 'all expenditure involved in acquiring fixed assets'. Running
expenses, or revenue expenditure, however, are those incurred in
'administering and carrying on the business'. Capital expenditure for
general practitioners, therefore, involves the provision of new capital
for buying something new, or replacing something which is worn
out or outdated. The capital cost is usually written off piecemeal year by
year for tax purposes. Running expenses are those which arise from the
day-to-day running of the practice. They are set against gross income
each year.

With recent changes in the tax laws the difference between these
two types of expenses has become more of theoretical than practical
importance. However, as most practice accounts are cast in this form,
it is important that a young doctor contemplating joining a practice
should be able to understand them.

In addition to practice expenses each general practitioner is liable to
income tax, National Insurance contributions and superannuation
contributions.

Running Expenses

The calculation of running expenses for doctors who work in private
premises differs from the calculation for those doctors who work in
health centres. In private premises all the expenses are met by the
general practitioners themselves. In health centres the cost of running
the health centres is initially met by the Area Health Authority which
charges the general practitioners using the centre rent and rates for the
rooms used and a percentage of the costs of running the centre as a
'service charge'.

A. Practice from Private Premises

The practice expenses of general practitioners who practise from private premises fall into four main categories.

1. Staff Costs

Wages of employed staff.
National Insurance contributions for employed staff.
Pension contributions for employed staff.

The conditions, hours and rates of pay for employed staff are determined by general practitioners themselves. If the staff are not related to the general practitioner or his partners, if they work more than five hours a week, *and* if they perform the qualifying duties laid down in the Red Book (para. 52.5), then 70 per cent of their wages will be reimbursed by the FPC up to a total of two full-time (or equivalent part-time) staff for each principal general practitioner who is in receipt of a basic practice allowance, provided that income from private practice is less than 10 per cent of practice income. A form ANC.1 has to be filled in for each qualifying member of staff on appointment and when any change is made in hours employed or wages paid. Claims for reimbursement are made to the FPC each quarter on forms ANC.2 and ANC.3.

National Insurance contributions for employed staff are paid, together with PAYE (Pay As You Earn) income tax deductions from staff salaries, direct to the local tax office each month. The form used and tables to enable the correct amount of PAYE to be calculated are supplied by the local tax office.

National Insurance contributions paid by general practitioners in respect of employed staff are reimbursed in full (52.8). Employers' contributions to certain staff pension schemes are also reimbursed (52.8, 52.9 and a later section in this chapter).

2. Cost of Premises

Rent of premises.
Rates for premises.
Repairs and redecorations.
Insurance of premises.

For premises rented from a private landlord, reimbursement of the rent is made by the Family Practitioner Committee provided that the District Valuer considers that the rent charged is appropriate. For premises owned by the partnership as a whole, or by one of the partners, a 'notional rent' as assessed by the District Valuer is paid. It may be a lengthy process for the practice and the District Valuer to agree an appropriate rent, but practitioners should continue the battle, by appeal if necessary, until a figure which they consider reasonable is obtained. An under-payment of £500 per year amounts to £5,000 in ten years. In case of difficulty advice may be sought from local colleagues and from the secretariat of the General Medical Services Committee through the local member.

Application for reimbursement of rent starts with a description of the premises on a form PREM.1 provided by the FPC. Thereafter quarterly payments are made by the FPC.

The rates for premises used by the practice have to be paid to the local council (as in any other business). Reimbursement of general and water rates (since April 1978) is made by the FPC when they receive evidence that they have been paid.

Redecorations and repairs cover the expenses involved in keeping the paintwork, furniture and fittings up to standard. The usual division of responsibility (which should be laid down in the lease) is that the landlord pays for external and structural repairs, while the practice is responsible for interior repairs and redecoration.

Insurance of premises and contents is the responsibility of the partners. As in any other property insurance a regular review is necessary to make sure that the insurance matches current value. Many partnerships also include insurance for consequential loss incurred in the event of fire or other disaster. Some include life or sickness policies on the partners' lives.

3. Servicing Costs

Telephones.
Heat and light.
Postage, stationery, printing.

These are inevitable costs and may be small or large depending on the amount of thought that has been put into the planning, the standards selected, and the extravagance or care with which the services are used.

4. Professional Costs

Accountancy.
Legal costs.
Bank charges.
Subscriptions.
Professional insurance.

Books and journals.

There are few general practitioners who understand the mysteries of accountancy, and there are few accountants who are experts in the intricacies of general practice finance. The process of mutual enlightenment proceeds slowly. Meanwhile the fees paid to an accountant who is versed in medical matters are often more than recovered by him annually through income tax saved.

Bank charges for practice overdrafts, unlike charges for private overdrafts, are allowed against tax and are considered in the income tax section.

Subscriptions to professional societies, such as the BMA or RCGP, may by partnership agreement be paid through the practice account, or may be paid by the individual doctor concerned. There is also an annual retention fee payable to the General Medical Council for retention of a practitioner's name on the Register.

Insurance for third-party risks is essential and prudence suggests that this should be a joint partnership responsibility. Another insurance which is essential for individual doctors is an insurance with a medical defence organisation. These organisations provide advice and legal defence for any member who is threatened with legal proceedings by a patient. It is usually a precondition of entering a partnership that a general practitioner should be so insured and that this insurance should be kept up to date.

Whether the purchase of books and journals is undertaken by the practice or by individual doctors is also a matter for partnership agreement. In view of the rising cost of books it would seem sensible to pool resources rather than risk duplication.

B. Practice from Health Centres

For those doctors who work in health centres there is a consolidated service charge levied by the Area Health Authority (Red Book para. 53.2) and deducted by the FPC from the quarterly payments. This charge covers staff costs, insurance of premises, telephone, heat and light, laundry, repairs and redecorations. It does not cover the employment of staff personally by the general practitioner or the renewal of personal medical equipment.

As the rent charged for the premises by the Area Health Authority is reimbursed by the Department of Health and Social Security through the Family Practitioner Committee, this transaction takes place above the head of the general practitioner as a book-keeping transaction from one government pocket to another. The proportion of the health centre rates which are payable by the general practitioner for the rooms his practice uses are similarly directly reimbursed. If the general practitioner in a health centre employs his own staff, he does so under the same terms and conditions as if he were in private accommodation.

The annual service charges are fixed by the Area Health Authority. It is usual for the general practitioners using the health centre to pay an agreed percentage of the total cost of running the health centre under each separate heading. For example, they might agree to pay 25 per cent of the wages of the cleaner, 20 per cent of heating and lighting costs, 50 per cent of the telephone rental and 100 per cent for the furniture in their consulting-rooms. The provisional charge for the current year is based on the latest known annual cost of running the centre. As the health centre accounts may be up to two years in arrears, the balancing charge to the general practitioners using the health centre may be considerable in these inflationary times.

If the practitioners think the percentage is unreasonably high, they may discuss the matter with the AHA. If after discussion practitioners are not satisfied with the assessment, they may ask for the matter to be referred to arbitration in accordance with paragraph 10 of the Model Health Centre Licence (Circular HC77/8 Appendix B) which was issued to all Area Health Authorities in April 1977.

Capital Expenses

Capital expenses are non-recurring. They are those which are involved in buying or building something new. Every purchase whether it be furniture, office equipment or medical equipment is technically a capital charge whether it is bought for the first time or is a replacement. Repairs to the practice premises are running expenses; building on an extension or converting a larder into a lavatory are capital expenses. The running costs of a car are a running expense, while the cost of buying a new car (although it may be in replacement of an old one) is a capital expense.

The capital expenses of running a practice depend almost entirely on the philosophy of the partners.

All Expenses

Many practices have in the past been ill-equipped and the standards accepted in waiting-rooms, offices and consulting-rooms have been lamentably low. It has taken general practitioners a long time to realise that the money that they as a profession spend on their practices as a legitimate expense is reimbursed to them through the 'expense factor' portion of their remuneration. This argument is developed in the last section of this chapter.

Although the expenses and proportions of expenses vary considerably from practice to practice, examination of the expenses for 1979 of various types of practice in South West England (health centre, private premises, single-handed, partnerships, city and rural) have shown variations within the following limits. There is no doubt that with wider sampling the differences between maximum and minimum costs would have been greater.

Table 9.1: Sample Costs per General Practitioner Principal in 1979

Type of expense	Minimum £	Maximum £
Wages of employed staff, including cleaning	2,780	6,256
Rent of Premises	180	4,100
Telephone	55	1,200
Heat and light	102	436
Stationery and printing	22	189
Postage	30	350
Accountancy and legal	70	410
Bank charges	Nil	260

After reimbursement of rent, rates and partial reimbursement of the salaries of ancillary staff have been included, the net total shared practice expenses range from £1,495 to £6,650 per general practitioner.

In addition to the expenses noted in Table 9.1, in most practices the partners themselves bear the other costs which are incurred because of their work. These include maintenance of a car or cars, the telephone answering service and telephones at their homes, the work their wives do for the practice, personal subscriptions and postgraduate course expenses. In 1979 these expenses might have amounted to over £4,500 per partner per year.

Obviously total practice expenses are related to the number of patients looked after by the practice. In the sample of practices analysed however, it was possible to calculate the practice expenses per patient, the income per patient, and the reimbursement. Although without a complete financial analysis of each practice it cannot be claimed that comparisons between practices are totally accurate, comparison between a sample high-expense practice (A) and a low-expense practice (B), both non-dispensing, is sufficiently interesting to be shown in Table 9.2.

Table 9.2: Comparison between a Sample High-expense and a Low-expense Practice

	1978	
	Practice A £	Practice B £
Gross expense per patient	5.86	3.64
Reimbursements	3.02	1.84
Net expense per patient	2.84	1.80
Gross income per patient	9.25	7.30
Net income per patient	6.41	5.50

Thus, in a high-spending practice, in which working conditions for doctors, staff and patients are considerably above average, the doctors took home almost £1 more per patient in 1978 than their colleagues in the low-spending practice. This apparent anomaly may be explained by the fact that the high-spending practice pays good wages to efficient staff, that there are call and recall systems not only for clinical conditions but also for those preventive procedures which attract item-of-service payments, that the forms for item-of-service payments are completed and forwarded promptly to the FPC. In addition a practice nurse is employed to whom appropriate procedures are delegated. The partners increase the practice income with part-time appointments (as described in Chapter 8).

Whether certain expenses should be borne by the practice, or personally by the partners, is a difficult question. It can only be decided by each partnership for itself. In some practices the expense of buying and running one car for each partner is borne by the practice. This has the advantage that if the purchase of a car results in an overdraft, a practice overdraft attracts tax relief whereas a private overdraft does not. On the other hand, in the past many general practitioners had cars that were expensive both to buy and run because 'it was on the practice'.

A similar question arises in the purchase of medical equipment. Most general practitioners buy their own personal medical equipment. For equipment or furniture which is more complicated and expensive it is essential that there should be a practice policy both for purchase and disposal. The partnership agreement should cover such matters to prevent misunderstandings and arguments.

Income Tax

By virtue of their independent-contractor status, general practitioners are self-employed. As such they are taxed under Schedule D for all payments received from the Family Practitioner Committee and many, but not all, of their other earnings. Under Schedule D all expenses incurred 'wholly and exclusively for professional purposes' are deducted from gross fees received to determine net taxable income.

Personal allowances, such as children's allowance, allowances for life insurance policies and wife's earned income allowance, are deducted from the net taxable income and income tax levied on the remainder. Thus the calculation for a single-handed general practitioner is simple:

a = income from FPC.
b = expenses of practice.
c = personal allowances.
d = taxable income.

$$a - (b + c) = d$$

Complicating factors are:

(1) Income from other sources from which tax has not been deducted (p).

(2) Income from other sources from which tax (t) has been deducted (q).

So the equation becomes: $a - (b + c) + p + q = d$

But when the tax on d has been determined (T) a certain amount has already been paid (t). So tax due = T − t.

This attempt to simplify matters may have confused some, but we hope it will have underlined how important it is, if a general practitioner has several sources of income, for the accountant to be informed of the exact amount earned from different sources and any tax paid under Schedule E (PAYE) or on tax paid shares, interest, or on building society interest, so that the assessment may be accurate. Any inaccuracies are more likely to be to the advantage of the income tax inspector than the general practitioner!

To make matters even more difficult when general practitioners practise in partnership it is the partnership which owes the tax on partnership income and not the individual practitioners.

The position is then calculated as follows:

Partners A: B: C
Personal allowances Ac Bc Cc
Total income of partnership I
Total expenses of partnership E
Personal practice expenses Ab Bb Cb
Tax payable by partnership = tax on $I - E - (Ac + Ab) - (Bc + Bb) - (Cc + Cb)$.

When the tax payable by the partnership has been determined it is divided between the partners according to their percentage of partnership income, minus (less) their personal allowances and expenses.

Having reached this stage, gentle reader, do not despair. For most general practitioners it will be sufficient to know the headings under which running and capital expenses can and should be claimed. A list of the running expenses allowable (to the extent that they are incurred in running the practice) can be found in Appendix G. This is a copy of an Appendix of the Report to the Conference of Local Medical Committees by the GMSC in 1976/7. If all general practitioners made sure that their accountants had a copy of this form, and they themselves made sure that they claimed all the expenses to which they were entitled, then the true expenses of running a practice would be reflected in the accounts.

For capital expenses involved in building something new or converting part of a building for practice purposes, there is no tax allowance. There is, however, an improvement grant scheme (para. 56.1 in the Red Book) which is discussed further in Chapter 4. It cannot be emphasised too strongly that the Family Practitioner Committee must approve the project *before* any contract is signed or work begun otherwise the grant will not be payable.

For the capital expense of buying new furniture or new equipment a capital allowance is made by the income tax authorities. Since 1972 the amount of the purchase price which can be set against tax in the year of purchase is up to 100 per cent at the discretion of the tax payer. If he does not choose to set the whole amount against tax in the first year, then the tax allowance in following years on the remainder is 25 per cent. The one exception to this ruling is the purchase of a car. When a car is purchased only 25 per cent of the price is allowed to be set against tax in the first year as it is in succeeding years.

Example: for a car which costs £4,000, 25 per cent (= £1,000) would be set against tax in the first year, i.e. the purchaser would not have to pay tax on £1,000 of his income. For the next year the 'written down' value of the car would be £3,000 and 25 per cent of this sum (i.e. £750) would be set against tax for that year. For the third year the written down value would be £2,250 and so on. If the car is sold at any time for more than the written down value, the tax authorities can claim back the excess part of the tax relief allowed in previous years. The last proviso applies not only to cars but also to sales of all capital equipment on which allowances have been claimed.

The running expenses of a car, which include not only petrol, oil, servicing, but repairs, licence and insurance, are allowed against tax annually – but a proportion (usually 10 per cent) is agreed with the tax authorities as being for private rather than professional use, and this proportion of the total expense is not allowed.

Lease or Buy?

Whether to rent furniture, equipment or cars, should be considered by partnerships and individual practitioners. The total cost of leasing and renting is allowed against tax as a running expense. If the purchase of an expensive item were to increase a personal overdraft (against the interest on which tax is not allowed) then it might be cheaper to lease than to buy. But no general rules apply, and each case must be worked out using the actual figures involved.

Special Points

1. Wife's Salary

The extent to which a general practitioner's wife takes part in the running of the practice varies enormously from practice to practice, from urban area to rural area. She may be a fully-fledged member of the practice staff, she may have very little connection with the practice. But however little or much she does it should be axiomatic that she is paid the rate for the job. If she is paid more than a certain amount per week (1980 £23.00) both she and her employer become liable for National Insurance contributions. In addition, if she earns more than £26.50 (1980) PAYE is deductible at source.

2. Doctor's Residence

Many general practitioners see patients at their own homes during the evenings and weekends they are on call. As recognition of the fact that the rooms in the house which may be used by patients have to be furnished, lit, and heated, it is customary for the tax authorities to allow a proportion of the expenses involved in running the doctor's house (rent, rates, repairs, heating, lighting, cleaning, and so on) to be set against income tax. Obviously in some practices this does not apply, but different inspectors may allow 25 per cent to 50 per cent of such costs to be set against income, according to the amount of use a doctor makes of his residence for these purposes. If a practitioner who claims part of the running expenses of his own home against his income tax sells his house at a profit he becomes liable to capital gains tax on that portion he has claimed against tax. If, however, he buys another house from which he is also going to practise in a similar way then the capital gain can be 'rolled over'. If this situation arises a practitioner should seek up-to-date advice from his accountant.

3. Bank Charges

Under the present regulations (1980) when the interest on a practice overdraft is allowed against tax but that on a personal overdraft is not, many young practitioners will find it advantageous to negotiate with their practice bank manager. Payment for all the work we do is in arrears—sometimes up to a year. In these circumstances most bank managers are willing to grant a practice overdraft, the limit depending on the practice net income. It would obviously be foolish to borrow so much that difficulties might arise. It is doubtful whether the bank manager would sanction it in any case. However, a practice overdraft of up to 10 per cent of the net income should not under any circumstances cause any embarrassment and could well be a help to a young practitioner entering practice.

National Insurance Contributions

There are four classes of National Insurance contributions. All general practitioner principals are required to pay Class 2 contributions (i.e. those for the self-employed). Most general practitioners will also be liable to pay Class 4 contributions as well. These are a supplement payable by the self-employed if their income is above a certain level. Some general practitioners, i.e. those who are employed part-time in other spheres, will also be liable to pay Class 1 contributions as employees. Fortunately, there is an overall limit to the contributions demanded, and practitioners are strongly advised to apply through their accountants for deferment or exemption if they have reasonable grounds for doing so.

National Insurance benefits are only related to the Class 2 contributions (self-employed) even if Class 1 payments are also made. Hence general practitioners working as employed persons (part-time) cannot claim the higher employed person's benefits even though they pay the higher contributions.

Superannuation

For general practitioners 6 per cent of the superannuable earnings received through the FPC are deducted at source. In this context 'superannuable earnings' means the total income received from the FPC minus a figure calculated to represent practice expenses. Contributions cease on retirement. The benefits which a general practitioner may receive under the scheme include:

(1) A lump sum, which is tax-free and payable on retirement.

(2) A retirement pension which is payable on retirement at 60 or after. It is paid from the age of 70 whether a general practitioner continues to work or not.

(3) An incapacity allowance and pension to a doctor who after five years' service has to retire owing to ill-health.

If a general practitioner dies in harness his family may receive:

(1) A death gratuity.
(2) A widow's pension.
(3) A child's allowance.

The pension which a general practitioner receives depends on the total of his superannuable earnings over his career within the National Health Service. The annual pension is 1.4 per cent (or about 1/70) of his total superannuable earnings. In 1972, in view of inflation, the Board of Inland Revenue agreed that each year's earnings should be 'dynamised'. Each year from 1948 to the present has been allocated a dynamising factor. The dynamising factor for 1960 to 1961 for example is 3.947. This means that in the calculation of total superannuable income, the sum credited to a general practitioner is the sum which he was informed was his superannuable pay in 1960 to 1961 multiplied by 3.947. In this way the pension earned by a general practitioner in his working life is not made obsolete by inflation.

The regulations concerning superannuation are exceedingly complex. If further information is needed the Department of Health and Social Security published a guide to the NHS Superannuation Scheme in 1974 which is available from Her Majesty's Stationery Office. A 'Practitioners' Supplement' to this guide was produced in 1977 and can be obtained from the DHSS Health Services Superannuation Division.

The General Medical Services Committee (further discussed in Chapter 15) negotiate the terms of general practitioners' superannuation and their secretariat can provide up-to-date information on request.

Staff Pensions

From April 1978 it became obligatory for an employer to offer each full-time employee either participation in the State Pension Scheme or participation in an approved private pension scheme. If prior to this a practitioner had arranged a private pension scheme for his staff then, provided the scheme and staff meet certain strict criteria (52.9), the employer's contributions, called 'qualifying superannuation contributions', are reimbursable in full on application to the FPC. There are two further important aspects to these regulations. Although no staff appointed to new posts are eligible, pension contributions for new staff appointed to take the place of staff who were eligible are reimbursable (52.9e). Secondly, increased contributions to the pension scheme in line with increases in salary are acceptable for reimbursement, provided they meet the criteria.

All contributions by employers to staff pension schemes should be entered as a practice expense for income tax purposes whether reimbursed or not.

Wider Implications

This chapter has of necessity been complicated. It has been hard going both to read and to write. Unfortunately, this turgidity reflects the complexity of the systems described—income tax, superannuation, and practice expenses in general.

But the importance of the subject to all general practitioners is undisputed. This is not only for personal reasons but because of the way in which the 'Practice Expense Factor' is calculated. Each year the Review Body, following representations by the BMA and the DHSS, fixes a target net income which they judge right at the time for the average general practitioner with an 'average' list to receive from the National Health Service. To this figure is added a sum to represent practice expenses. The total cake (target net income plus expense factor for all the general practitioners in the country) is then divided into its various slices (capitation fees, basic practice allowance, and so on).

Each year the Review Body decides by how much each portion of each general practitioner's income will be altered (e.g. £200 on basic practice allowance, 10p on cervical smears) in order to attain the overall expenditure (i.e. total cake) they consider fair.

The 'Expense Factor' for 1980/1 was fixed at £6,850 for each general practitioner in April 1980. This figure is calculated by taking a representative sample of the most recent income tax returns of general practitioners throughout the country. To this figure is added a 'best-guess', a sum to make up for inflation, since the returns were made. But the basis of the Expense Factor is the expenses actually incurred by practitioners and declared to the income tax authorities. The system is such that if every general practitioner in the sample equipped himself to the hilt, bought an ECG machine, and employed as many skilled ancillary staff as he thought he needed, then these expenses would be reflected in the expense factor within five years, and would be reimbursed to *all* general practitioners.

The authors believe that many general practitioners, including no doubt some of those whose tax returns are sampled, do not claim in full the expenses to which they are entitled. This affects not only the amount of tax which those general practitioners themselves pay, but also diminishes the Expense Factor—and therefore the income that *all* general practitioners receive.

It is in the interest of the whole profession that all general practitioners should have an accurate working knowledge of their practice expenses, and that the practice accounts should reflect these expenses in full.

Further Reading

BMA. *Members' Handbook*, Section V: Superannuation (BMA, 1977).
Practitioners' supplement to the *Guide on National Health Service Superannuation for England and Wales.* DHSS Health Services Superannuation Division (Hesketh House, 200/220 Broadway, Fleetwood, Lancs).
Report of the General Medical Services Committee to the Annual Conference of Representatives of Local Medical Committees 1977. Appendix II: Memorandum on Practice Expenses (BMA, 1977).

10 PRACTICE ACCOUNTS AND ANALYSIS

For most aspiring partners and often for established partners practice accounts and balance sheets are a mystery. Such a balance sheet, however, is the sole objective way of comparing the financial state of the practice from one year to the next. It is the only factual way of comparing the financial arrangements of two different practices. Unless partners understand how to interpret their practice accounts they are unable to relate feelings to facts, or to take action to correct losses of income due to poor organisation.

Practice Accounts

Although there are differences in presentation between one accountant and another all practice accounts should include the following components:

(1) Statement of capital assets at the beginning and end of the year.
(2) Statement of outstanding credits owed to the practice on the last day of the year.
(3) The bank balance in the practice account at the end of the year.
(4) Statement of outstanding debts owed by the practice on the last day of the year.
(5) Income due to individual partners during the year according to the practice agreement.
(6) Income received by individual partners during the financial year.

These figures enable calculation to be made of:

(7) The total net assets (or debits) of the practice at the end of the year.
(8) The amount by which individual partners have underdrawn or overdrawn according to the partnership agreement.
(9) A profit and loss account, showing the gross income, expenses and net profit.

In order to clarify these points a sample balance sheet is shown (Figure 10.1) for a three-man practice in 1978, with the figures

Figure 10.1: Sample Practice Balance Sheet

DRS A, B AND C
BALANCE SHEET AS AT 31ST DECEMBER 1978

1977			
	FIXED ASSETS		
3,241	Surgery and office equipment at cost or value introduced	3,313	(1)
1,190	Less: depreciation to date	1,508	(2)
2,051		1,805	(3)
	CURRENT ASSETS		
529	Debtors and Prepayments	560	(4)
536	Balance at Bank	984	(5)
25	Cash in Hand	25	(6)
1,090		1,569	(7)
	LESS: CURRENT LIABILITIES		
—	Income tax	1,224	(8)
1,171	Creditors and accrued expenses	971	(9)
		2,195	(10)
(81)	NET CURRENT LIABILITIES	(626)	(11)
£1,970	NET ASSETS	£1,179	(12)

REPRESENTED BY PARTNERS' CAPITAL ACCOUNTS

	Dr A	Dr B	Dr C	
Balance at 1.1.78	578	(218)	1,610	(13)
Profit for year	13,605	13,201	8,881	(14)
	14,183	12,983	10,491	(15)
Less — Drawings	12,785	12,693	11,000	(16)
	£ 1,398	£ 290	£ (509)	(17)

£1,970			£1,179	(18)

We have prepared, without carrying out an audit, the above Balance Sheet as at 31st December 1978, and annexed Profit and Loss Account for the year ended on that date from the accounting records of our client and from information and explanations supplied to us.

Mole House
The Wood
Exeter

Snooks Bloggs and Co.
Chartered Accountants

4th July 1979

discussed under the headings as in 1 to 9 above.

Capital Assets

These are shown on the balance sheet as 'surgical and office equipment at cost or value introduced' under the heading FIXED ASSETS. It includes the total value of the equipment owned by the practice, e.g. carpets, curtains, desks, chairs, filing cabinets, medical equipment. In practices which own their premises it will also include these at valuation. At the beginning of 1978 the figure in the sample balance sheet was £3,313 (line 1). The comparable figure for 1977 was £3,241 from which can be calculated the fact that £72 of capital equipment was bought during the year. The figure of £1,508 (line 2) is the cumulative depreciation which has occurred since the assets were acquired, so that the figure of £1,805 (line 3) is the total written-down value of the fixed assets owned by the practice at the end of 1978.

Outstanding Credits

These are listed under the heading of CURRENT ASSETS. They include items which are due to the practice for work carried out during the year for which payment is received after the year end (debtors), and pre-payments—which are estimates of payments made in advance for such items as rent, insurances and rates. It will be noted that this figure for debtors and prepayments of £560 (line 4) is far too low to include reimbursement of rents, rates and the 70 per cent of staff salaries paid out in the last quarter of 1978 and not received until well on into 1979. Because many items of NHS practice income are paid in arrears and are difficult for the accountant to estimate, receipts for such items are usually counted as income during the year in which they are received. When analysing practice accounts this does not matter provided that a consistent policy is followed. If these payments are included in 'year earned' one year and 'year received' in another this can produce considerable distortion in apparent profits.

The bank balance, on the last day of the year is entered, if in credit, under current assets. If in debt it is entered under current liabilities.

Outstanding Debts

These are the debts incurred by the practice during the year but unpaid on the day the books closed. They are listed under the heading CURRENT LIABILITIES. The figure of £971 quoted for 'creditors and accrued expenses' (line 9) is composed of items such as PAYE for staff (incurred but not paid), bills for professionals (e.g. accountants) who present their bills in arrears, estimated outstanding accounts for telephones and electricity.

Figures provided under the above headings enable the financial state of the practice on the last day of the year to be stated. In the example given the outstanding debts (line 10), which includes £1,224 unpaid income tax (line 8), exceed the outstanding credits (line 7) by £626 (line 11). Subtraction of this figure from that for the written-down fixed assets (line 4) gives the net assets of the practice at the year end as £1,179 (line 12).

Income Due to Individual Partners

These figures are calculated by dividing the net practice income for the year in the proportions for individual partners as set out in the partnership agreement. In the example quoted the sum to be distributed was £35,687. In this practice each partner keeps his own seniority allowance, the balance of the profit being divided in a way which reflects the agreed workload of the partners. Division in this way resulted in the money due to partner A being £13,605, partner B £13,201 and partner C £8,881. These figures are presented in the balance sheet under 'Profit for year' (line 14). The calculation is usually presented to the partners by the accountant on a separate page of the accounts called 'Division of profits for the year 19 . .'.

Income Received by Partners. These figures are noted in the balance sheet under the heading of 'drawings' (line 16) and amounted to £12,785 for partner A, £12,693 for partner B and £11,000 for partner C. This is the money which the individual partners received from the practice during the year.

In the accounts of the sample practice there is a difference between the amount of money each partner received (drawings, line 16) and the amount he should have received according to the practice agreement (profit, line 14). The reason is that in this practice the income tax on the partnership is paid by the practice as a whole. As the three partners have different tax liabilities within this sum (see Chapter 9) and the practice cheques to the tax authorities contain payment in equal shares, the differences have to be corrected the following year when the tax position has been calculated. In the sample accounts the line 'balance at 1.1.78' (line 13) shows that the position at the beginning of 1978 was that partner A was owed £578, partner C was owed £1,610, while partner B had been overpaid by £218. Correction of this and payment of tax during 1978 resulted in the position that by the end of 1978 Dr A was owed £1,398, Dr B was owed £290 and Dr C owed the practice £509 (line 17). These figures will appear on the 1979 accounts as 'balance at 1.1.79' in line 13, to be corrected the following year.

Profit and Loss Account

This account presents on the one hand the gross income received by the practice over the year, on the other a list of expenses incurred. The net profit of the partnership for the year is calculated by subtracting expenses from gross income. This figure forms the basis of the calculation of the income due to each of the partners. Some practices use the model expense form produced by the GMSC and reproduced in Appendix G. Certainly practices which do not use this form would be well advised to check their profit and loss account against it to make sure that they and their accountants are not overlooking expenses which can legitimately be claimed.

Practice Finance Analysis

Reference has been made in Chapters 8 and 9 to the need for analysis of income and expenditure. The point was made that unless the partners had some idea of the income generated by their various activities they had few facts to rely upon when deciding whether to expand or contract in any particular direction. A simple example would be the decision whether to give influenza vaccines after issuing a prescription which the patient would exchange at the chemist, or whether to buy the vaccine in bulk and claim payment from the FPC (under para. 44.13 of the Red Book). In the first instance no profit or loss is made. In the second the result will depend on the efficiency with which the business side is organised – buying more vaccine than is used, delay in presenting the accounts to the FPC or failure to account for all the injections given may all result in financial loss instead of the expected small profit. It is only by looking at the final figures that the partners can decide whether it is financially better for them to buy their own vaccine the following year or to issue patients with prescriptions.

The ability to make such an analysis depends on keeping accurate books for both income and expenditure. It is a simple matter to buy one book for each. These are laid out with a column for the date on the left. In the next column is shown the source of income or the item of expenditure. In the third column is the amount. The succeeding columns are headed by the classified source of income, or the classified type of expenditure. The headings chosen will vary according to the

Figure 10.2: Sample Income Analysis Book

Date	Source	Amount	Paid to Bank	Insurance Medicals Reports	Cremation Fees	Private Patients	Outside Appointments Nat. Child. Home	IBA	Fire Service	Devon CC AHA DHSS	Sundries
1977											
Feb 2	Conway and Stewart re P. Russell	5.50		5.50							
10	Legal and General (P. Cradock)	4.30		4.30							
10	Devon and Cornwall Police re Taylor	5.00								5.00	
23	G.C. Allen Pole	4.00	18.80			4.00					

Figure 10.3: Sample Expenditure Analysis Book

Date 1977	Paid to	Amount	Salaries Staff Trainee	PAYE NI	Rent Rates	Postage	Printing Stationery Office Equip.	Light Heat Telephone	Renewals Repairs	Profess. Charges	Sundries
May 30	Rotadex	27.22					27.22				
June 5	Inland Revenue PAYE	455.99		455.99							
	Inland Revenue NI	211.74		211.74							
	Dr A.B.C.	32.00	32.00								
	SWEB	17.43						17.43			

circumstances of individual practices. Figure 10.2 shows possible headings for an income analysis book; Figure 10.3 for an expenditure analysis, together with a few sample entries.

The samples quoted in the figure do not show either direct credits in the income analysis or standing orders in the expenditure analysis. Direct credits include all the money transferred directly to the partners account. Examples are the quarterly payments made to the practice by the FPC, or direct payments for part-time salaried employment undertaken by one or more of the partners (e.g. school medical officer, industrial work). Standing orders may include payments to partners or staff, payments for furniture or books by arrangement. In some practices these payments are included in the analysis as they occur. Many practices, however, find it more convenient to list these separately and include them in the final analysis at the year end.

Full analysis of income includes not only broad categories of payment but also further subdivision. In order to do this it is necessary to look in more detail at the notification of income received quarterly from the Family Practitioner Committee. The total amount will appear on the bank balance as a single entry directly credited to the partnership four times a year with subsidiary credits for reimbursements or maternity services at other times. But on each occasion that the FPC transmits such a sum the practice receives a statement on which analysis has already been made as to the source of income. It is a simple matter for whoever is carrying out the analysis to add up the sums on the four statements received for carrying out individual services to give an annual total. In this way the income received from different sources for all the activities carried out by the partners can be calculated on an annual basis. By similarly using the expenditure analysis book the expenses of the practice can also be calculated on an annual basis. In Appendix H one method of itemising these analyses is illustrated. By analysing income and expenditure in this way comparison can be made with previous years and with the national figures.

There is no doubt that such analysis takes time and effort. Unless commensurate benefits are received many general practitioners will not bother to initiate them. There are several factors to be considered. First, the salary of a financial secretary is eligible for 70 per cent reimbursement. In our experience such a secretary can comfortably look after the financial affairs of a three-partner practice on a part-time basis. Her duties need not be carried out in surgery hours. Much of her work can be carried out at home. Again it is our experience that this is a job which married ex-bank employees with young families find both challenging and interesting.

As regards benefits the increase in fees from cervical cytology tests alone paid for a large part of the non-reimbursed salary of a financial secretary in one of our practices. Analysis clearly showed that although the tests were being carried out only a small proportion of the fees was being claimed. In another practice which had been under the impression that its immunisation programme was adequate, financial analysis resulted in a fresh look and reorganisation of the system.

Such financial analysis within a practice presents various topics for discussion between partners. The exercise becomes even more interesting when different practices compare figures. At a recent course on practice management during which principals from different practices produced comparable figures, the income per patient per year from immunisation procedures varied in different practices from 2p to 56p, a difference of 2,800 per cent. There is no doubt in our minds that the employment of a secretary who produces an annual analysis of income and expenditure for discussion by the partners and staff is a major advance in rationalisation of practice management.

Over the past ten years the amount of money invested in a practice has increased out of all recognition. For those in their own premises the capital value of the buildings has in many cases trebled. With inflation and amalgamation the gross incomes of practices have increased dramatically. In many cases expenses have increased even more dramatically.

Whether we like it or not, general practitioners are in business. Balance sheets and analyses of costs and of income are the tools of business just as much as the stethoscope is a tool for the practice of medicine. It is both foolish and expensive to work in the dark.

PART FIVE: PAPERS

11 THE PRACTICE AND THE LAW

Introduction

Becoming a principal in general practice involves undertaking formal relationships with many different organisations and people. They include:

(a) A contract with the Family Practitioner Committee.
(b) A contract with individual patients.
(c) A contract with partners.
(d) A contract with each employee.
(e) Contracts with landlords (or, for those working in owner-occupied premises, mortgages and/or loan agreements).
(f) Contracts with insurance companies.

(a) The Contract with the Family Practitioner Committee

Many doctors find it difficult to understand what is meant by 'independent contractor'. In fact, it is the common state for most senior professionals, and only since the National Health Service led to the introduction of salaried consultants in 1948 was the situation altered. Until that time most doctors, lawyers and accountants were self-employed independent contractors offering their services in return for a fee. For general practitioners, that situation continues except that the Secretary of State for Health and Social Security has underwritten the patient's obligation to pay a fee. The significance and consequences of the independent-contractor status for general practice and general practitioners have been further discussed in Chapter 2.

When he signs his contract with a Family Practitioner Committee on becoming a principal, the general practitioner states the area in which he is to practise, the premises from which he intends to practise, the hours available for consultation, and the name and address of any other doctor with whom he intends to practise. He agrees to provide certain services (general medical, maternity, contraceptive). The regulations lay down that these shall be 'necessary and appropriate personal medical services of the type usually provided by general

practitioners'. In return for providing these services he is entitled to
National Health Service fees and allowances.

(b) The Contract with the Patient

Each person is issued with a National Health Service medical card
(FP.4). This card forms the basis of a tripartite contract; a contract
between the patient and the doctor in which the doctor agrees to
provide services, and a contract between the doctor and the Family
Practitioner Committee acting as the agent of the Area Health Authority
in which the latter contracts to pay the doctor the current fees as laid
down in the Red Book. On his part, the doctor contracts with the
Family Practitioner Committee that he will fulfil the terms and conditions of service regarding the provision of medical services as far as
that particular patient is concerned. The contract between the doctor
and the patient is therefore a personal one, just as the relationship
between the doctor and his patient is also personal.

Most patients who join a doctor's list present the doctor with their
medical cards. Some will not be able to find their medical cards. These
patients should be given a form (FP.1) which they complete and present
in place of a medical card. When patients register the birth of newly
born infants they are given a small pink card (FP.58) by the Registrar
of Births and Deaths which fulfils the same purpose as a medical card.
This is given to the doctor when he accepts the infant on his list.

When patients present the doctor or his receptionist with their
medical card it is important to check that they have completed and
signed either Parts A or B of the card. When a new patient registers
many practices use the opportunity to provide a practice information
leaflet giving details of surgery times and special clinics together with
other general information about the practice to the new patients.
Some doctors like to see all their new patients, partly to emphasise
the personal nature of the doctor/patient relationship, but often also
to record basic background information on a medical record card.

Once the medical card has been received by the doctor or his
receptionist, the doctor must sign the card and date it. This signifies
his acceptance of the patient on his list. He should also enter whether
or not he is to supply drugs to the patient. If he is entitled to claim
rural practice payments then he should enter the mileage in the space
provided. The completed card is then sent to the Family Practitioner
Committee.

(c) The Contract with Partners

There is nothing quite like a happy partnership. Doctors in such a group know that they do not need formal agreements to keep them happy; but sensible general practitioners know that when things go wrong a properly drawn partnership deed can save distress and embarrassment to everyone.

No one should enter into partnership anticipating trouble. Ideally, a partnership should be a progressive association of colleagues and friends, but agreed rules at the start may help determine how the relationships develop and can determine what happens if they break down. It is much easier to draw up the governing rules of the partnership before rather than after the partnership begins. It is better still to have them written in legal form from the start. However, solicitors work at their own speed and often formal deeds cannot be prepared in time to meet the start of the partnership. If the rules are agreed, an exchange of letters of intent between the doctors involved and their solicitors is usually a satisfactory guarantee, provided the letters also include a date by which the partnership documents must be signed.

Which Solicitor?

Most solicitors are prepared to draw up partnership agreements but some are much more experienced in this work than others. Frequently, medical groups will ask solicitors used to preparing medical partnership deeds to act for them. The Personal Services Bureau of the BMA issues an advisory leaflet on partnership agreements (Medical Partnerships under the National Health Service) and is willing to inspect members' draft agreements and advise on them.

How Much Does it Cost?

A properly drawn partnership agreement is not a cheap document, and may cost several hundred pounds. In the event of later disagreement it can save many thousands of pounds.

What is Covered?

The agreement should cover every aspect of doctors working together, the rules governing both the day-to-day working of the practice and long-term practice policy. It should specify the arrangements for the medical policy and management of the practice as well as the appointment of staff.

It should set out how the rota for on-call, holidays, sick leave and study leave is drawn up, and must lay down rules covering the financial arrangements for the practice — not only where money earned comes from (and what exactly is partnership money) but how and when shares are paid to individual doctors. Financial clauses should cover such things as tax liability, ownership of partnership property (both freehold and leasehold), liability for rented accommodation, and the capital assets of the firm.

The arrangements for retirement must be agreed, and the procedure to be followed in case of the death or chronic illness of a partner stated. It is essential to set out how and for what reasons the partnership may be dissolved. The more comprehensive the partnership deed the more it is likely to cost *but* in the event of disagreement between partners, the easier the solution.

The following is a check list covering items which appear in most partnership deeds:

(1)   *Who?* Who are to form the medical partnership? What is its name?

(2)   *When?* When does it start, how long may it continue? Does anyone have a fixed date or age of retirement?

(3)   *Where?* Where does the medical partnership practise, is there a defined area?

(4)   *What?* What notice must a partner give if he wishes to leave?

(5)   *Holidays.* How many days (or weeks) are allowed each year? Who has first choice (or is it by rota?)

(6)   *Study and Sabbatical Leave.* These need to be specified.

(7)   *Sick Leave.* Sick leave rights need to be stated since ill-health of one partner throws both an increased workload and an increased financial burden on the remaining partners. Must partners have an agreed minimum sickness insurance? Who pays for it, the partnership or the individual doctor? Who gets it? Who pays for a locum if needed? What is the partnership policy with regard to money received under the National Health Service sickness benefit scheme? How long will the partnership allow a sick member to continue as a partner?

(8)   *Money In.* It is essential to specify precisely what constitutes 'partnership money' and what is the individual doctor's own money. For example, does every professional fee go to the partnership (what about lecture fees earned on a partner's half-day or weekend off or money earned during holidays)? How is the scale of private fees of the partnership determined? What is a *Gift* and what is a 'payment for professional service'? What about legacies, are these ever equivalent to

professional receipts? Seniority and vocational training payments are individually earned by a doctor, but are they to go into the partnership pool or not? If they are, who is to benefit from the superannuation which goes with them, the individual who earned them or everyone?

(9) *Money Out.* Which bank holds the partnership accounts and who signs the cheques? What expenses are to be met by the partnership and how is the remainder to be divided? Is there to be immediate parity for a new partner, or is this to be gradually attained? What about car expenses and telephone expenses?

(10) *Accountancy.* How is income and expenditure to be recorded, what are the accounting days and who is to prepare the partnership accounts?

(11) *On Duty and Off Duty.* How is the partnership's National Health Service practice preserved (e.g. no partner may withdraw from night or week-end duty, and no partner may do anything to prejudice his receipt of a basic practice allowance)? Are equal shares to be paid for equal work? Do senior (or older) partners drop money when they drop duty?

(12) *Precedence.* Do senior partners have privileges and, if so, what are they and are these reasonable?

(13) *Partnership Meetings.* Are these to be held regularly? How is the chairman appointed, and does the post rotate amongst all partners? Are minutes to be kept?

(14) *Administration.* What management jobs are to be allocated to partners (e.g. finance, staffing, building and maintenance) and do they rotate?

(15) *Miscellaneous.*

    (a) Where may partners live?

    (b) If a partner moves, who pays increased telephone costs? (e.g. for an extended direct line from the practice switchboard).

    (c) If a partner leaves, must he covenant not to set up in opposition practice within a defined area? How much does he pay if he breaks this covenant?

    (d) Is there an agreed selection procedure for new partners?

    (e) Should there be a clause covering arbitration where partners fail to agree, e.g. over the valuation of freehold property when a retiring partner is leaving?

    (f) Representative appointments (service on the LMC etc.) are often looked upon as a responsibility (and honour) for the practice. Is the serving partner to be covered during his absence by the remaining partners?

(g) Outside appointments are quite common. What is the practice policy in respect of new appointments? Does the agreement need to refer to this? Can a partner give up an existing appointment without the consent of his partners (practice income may fall)?

(h) Is it necessary to have a special rule to cover the possibility of a partner being called up for National Service in Her Majesty's Armed Forces?

(i) Is membership of the Medical Defence Union or Medical Protection Society or a similar organisation obligatory?

(j) Are partners allowed to engage in other businesses (e.g. can one become a farmer)?

(k) Does the agreement specifically state that personal debts may not be secured against partnership assets (without the written consent of all the partners)?

(16) It is usual for the deed to state that 'all shall employ themselves diligently in the practice and use their utmost endeavours' and go on to state that 'each shall be faithful and just one to the other'. Finally, all agree to share the cost of the preparation of the deed.

Clearly, legal documents—however comprehensive and however pious the clauses—cannot make a medical partnership work. It is the spirit with which each doctor enters into partnership which ensures success or failure.

(d) The Contract with Staff

In some practices each doctor has an individual secretary/receptionist who gets to know the working habits, outside commitments and rate of consultation of her particular doctor. This makes for a good working relationship but has the disadvantage of producing problems during holidays, sickness and other leave. It also presumes that the secretary is going to be available all day for that particular doctor. A more efficient system for the average practice is to try and make all reception staff virtually interchangeable so that they can all receive patients, take telephone calls and file records at various times. If this system is used then there should still be one member of staff who does most of the secretarial work with another member of staff to back her up in the case of her absence. For each employee a job description should be part of her contract.

The terms of service of staff will depend on the needs of the practice, but for part-time staff, hourly rates of pay are usual. These should be reviewed annually and incremental increases in line with nationally accepted norms considered. Guidance for rates of pay for secretaries and nurses can be obtained by reference to comparable hospital or health authority rates. Sick leave and holiday arrangements vary from practice to practice, but it is usual for most staff to have three to four weeks' paid holiday.

It is a good principle to pay good staff well. Reception staff who are well trained and can deal correctly with patients should be highly valued. Their cost to the doctors is small when weighed against the beneficial effect they have on the practice. Moreover the 30 per cent of their salaries which is not reimbursed is tax deductible.

When appointing new staff it should be made quite clear to them what their hours will be, any holiday relief work expected, their rate of pay, number of weeks' holiday and sick-leave allowance. Above all the importance of confidentiality of information should be emphasised. A gossiping receptionist can soon damage the practice's reputation.

For further training of staff, the Association of Medical Secretaries may be helpful. This organisation holds local meetings and annual symposia. Doctors may consider taking their staff with them to medical meetings in practice organisation, and for reading material an introductory book is *The Medical Secretary's Handbook* by Michael Drury (1975).

Contracts of Employment for Staff

Since the Employment Protection Act of 1975 each employer has had specific obligations to his employees. This Act affects every practitioner, even if he only employs one person. The rights and obligations involved are as follows:

1. Particulars of Employment. The Act lays down that particulars of the contract of employment must be given in writing to all employees with three exceptions:

(a) Where the employee is the husband or wife.

(b) Where an employee engaged since 1 January 1976 is employed for less than 16 hours per week.

(c) Where an employee who had by then worked for five years continuously is employed for less than eight hours per week.

The particulars, which can be given by letter or in any other written form, must include (a) salary, (b) job title, (c) holiday entitlement, (d) sick leave and pay, (e) period of notice, (f) right to redundancy payment, (g) rights against unfair dismissal, (h) right of union membership, (i) disciplinary rules and (j) grievance procedure.

2. Itemised Pay Statement. The employer must itemise his employee's pay statement so that it shows gross wages or salary, deductions (and for what purposes they are made) and the net pay.

3. Notice. After four weeks of continuous employment, an employee can be dismissed only by notice so that a practitioner must decide in that initial period whether to dismiss an employee summarily.

Between the four weeks' qualifying period and 24 months of continuous employment, one weeks' notice of termination of employment must be given. After two years, the employee is entitled to one week's notice for each completed year of employment up to a maximum of twelve weeks.

Notice should always be given in writing.

4. Dismissal. Every person who has been employed for a minimum of 26 weeks has a right not to be unfairly dismissed, subject to there being a minimum number of employees in the business (currently four). If an employee is unsatisfactory, he or she must be given a proper warning and an opportunity to improve. If things are still unsatisfactory, a final warning in writing must be given. If there seems to be no alternative to dismissal, the employee must be given a proper opportunity to state his or her case and can then be given written notice of termination. The employee can call upon the employer to give a written statement of reasons for dismissal though, in practice, it is advisable to incorporate the reasons in the notice of dismissal.

An aggrieved employee can apply to an Industrial Tribunal for compensation to be paid by the employer. Resignation as an alternative to dismissal counts as dismissal and enables a disgruntled employee to take proceedings.

5. Maternity. Associated with the general right against unfair dismissal are a female employee's additional rights:

(a) Not to be dismissed because of pregnancy without being first offered suitable alternative employment.

(b) To be given six weeks' maternity pay provided she works until eleven weeks before her estimated date of confinement and has at that time completed two years' continuous service.

(c) To return to her job within 29 weeks of confinement.

6. Redundancy. A person who has been employed for a minimum of 104 weeks and who is dismissed because of cessation of business (such as closure of a practice) is entitled to a redundancy payment calculated according to a statutory formula. The employer can claim rebate of one half of the sum paid from the State Redundancy Payment Fund, and the balance (or a proportion of the balance if the member of staff is employed only partly on qualifying duties) from the Family Practitioner Committee.

7. Liability for Accidents at Work. All employers are liable for accidents to employees caused by defective equipment, leaving the employer in appropriate cases to claim an indemnity from the manufacturer. Employers must also insure against claims by employees for accidents occurring to them in the course of their work.

8. Sex Discrimination. An employer must not discriminate against a married or unmarried person of either sex in the arrangements he makes for determining who will be offered employment. There are separate provisions relating to advertising. A practitioner must distinguish between applicants for a job by their ability only and should in advertising make it clear that a post is open to members of either sex.

9. Equal Pay. Men and women in the same employment must be treated equally in terms of pay so long as the woman's and the man's work are of the same nature in terms of effort, skill and decision. This applies, for instance, to a practice employing two part-time managers, one a man and one a woman, in that if their duties are comparable they must be paid equally.

10. Union Membership. An employee is entitled to belong to a Trade Union and to take part in its activities outside working hours without interference from the employer.

(e) Contract with Landlords or Mortgagor

Most doctors will either rent their practice accommodation (and have a contract with a landlord) or own their premises.

In the case of doctors in rented premises, the landlord may either be the Area Health Authority or an independent private landlord.

The Model Health Centre licence (sent by the Department of Health and Social Security to all Area Health Authorities in April 1977) forms a basis on which doctors who practise from health centres may make a contract with the Area Health Authority.

Contracts with private landlords are individually arranged. Good legal advice is essential when drawing up such a contract.

General practitioners who work from their own premises usually have a mortgage or a loan from either the General Practice Finance Corporation or from a Building Society. In either case, a further contract is inevitable. A fuller description of the methods of financing premises and the agreements required is given in Chapter 4.

(f) Contracts Covering Insurance

Apart from life insurance and mortgage protection, general practitioners as independent contractors need to insure themselves against claims from staff or patients who may be injured on the practice premises. These are termed Employer's Liability and Public Liability insurance. In addition, a doctor's full insurance against medical malpractice is essential and should be a condition of joining a partnership.

General practitioners have full-time responsibility for patient care. They have particular need for insurance against absence through sickness, especially since the sickness of a partner may entail the employment of a locum practitioner. Some companies are prepared to give permanent sickness cover specially adapted to the needs of doctors in partnership. It is usual for partners to insure also against consequential loss through general insurances covering the practice premises and contents.

Insurance is such an important subject that most general practitioners will need specialist advice. The services of an insurance broker used to dealing with the needs of family doctors may be useful, or advice from the Medical Insurance Agency or the Medical Sickness Annuity and Life Assurance Society Limited should be sought.

Breaking Contracts

No one really enters into a contract with the object of breaking it.

However, for all sorts of reasons it is sometimes necessary to terminate contracts. All legal agreements should have a clause which clearly sets out the procedure to be followed if the contract is to be terminated. It is as well to be aware of the rules when entering into a contract.

If the delicate relationship between doctor and patient is broken, the contract which the doctor entered into with the Family Practitioner Committee and the patient will have to be ended. There is a set procedure for doing this.

The doctor may notify the FPC that he wishes a certain patient to be removed from his list and, provided the patient is not under medical treatment at the time, the patient is removed from the practitioner's list after seven days. The doctor does not have to give reasons for his request.

The patient has similar rights. He may inform the FPC that he wishes to be removed from the doctor's list (or change to another doctor). With the written consent of his doctor he may change immediately to another practitioner, provided the second practitioner agrees, otherwise he must give fourteen days' notice of his decision to be removed from his doctor's list.

We believe that the doctor has a duty to his patient to consider whether or not the breakdown in relationships is a symptom of the patient's ill-health and, if so, whether or not steps to heal the breach would be more in keeping with the proper role of the practitioner. Only in the very last resort should doctors remove patients from their list. It is an admission of failure but it happens occasionally to all of us.

Disciplinary Procedure

Occasionally, following a breakdown in relations between a doctor and his patient, a complaint is made. This complaint is made to the Family Practitioner Committee by the patient. It may be formal or informal.

In the case of formal complaints there is a medical service procedure which has to be followed. All principals in general practice should be aware of the complaints procedure which patients may use against them. No one enters practice contemplating being subject to disciplinary procedure, but it can happen unexpectedly.

The commonest cause of complaint is 'failure to visit' and doctors who have been subject to this complaint often wonder why it happened; usually the reason is a failure in communication between doctor and patient. The doctor who may have said on the telephone, 'I think the problem is so and so and if you do such and such, the situation will improve'—may have meant to add, 'If it doesn't, let me know and I'll come,' but this has been construed by the patient as 'doctor refused to come'. Hence the complaint.

The Administrator (or his deputy) and the Chairman of the Family Practitioner Committee will usually try and sort out most complaints informally. They will try to find out what each side thinks happened and then try to settle the matter amicably between the parties concerned. If the complaint is apparently serious, or the complaining patient or doctor demands a formal hearing, then the Administrator of the Family Practitioner Committee must arrange for a hearing before the Medical Services Committee.

The procedure of a medical services committee is complicated and currently (1980) under review. For detailed advice and information the doctor is advised to contact his medical defence organisation. Both the Medical Defence Union and the Medical Protection Society publish advisory booklets which members receive on request.

Further Reading

Complaints to Family Practitioner Committees (Medical Defence Union, London, 1975).
Law and the Doctor (Medical Defence Union, London, 1977).
Medical Partnerships under the National Health Service (BMA Personal Services Bureau, 1976).
Pitfalls and Worries of the Young Doctor (Medical Protection Society, London).
Professional Conduct and Discipline (General Medical Council, London, 1977).

12 RECORDS

Record-keeping has always been one of the weaker aspects of general practice. Even now many general practitioners maintain that they can practise good medicine without writing in the patient's notes, relying on their memory and relationship with the patient. It is only over the past twenty years, with the example set by doctors such as Keith Hodgkin and John Fry, that interest has been stimulated in this field so that some new form of record-keeping seems to be reported every few months. Even as recently as 1972 Dawes surveyed eight practices and considered the data recorded to be of poor quality. In 50 per cent of episodes no diagnosis was entered, in 10 per cent a diagnosis was recorded without supporting evidence. Less than half contained information about symptoms. Physical signs were only mentioned in one third of cases.

A general practitioner must be quite clear in his own mind why he is keeping a record of his consultation. At the simplest level it may be to remind himself of what he has prescribed next time he sees the patient. However, there are other important reasons for keeping good records:

(1) In a partnership it is vital that other partners know what has been happening to the patient, as they may be called upon when the patient's doctor is not available. Some practices share patients freely between partners.

(2) Records should contain details of on-going events such as immunisation schedules and results of cervical smears, so that a course of action may be followed through logically.

(3) Any doctor referring to the records should be able to identify previous episodes of importance in the patient's past medical history, be able to continue management on a day-to-day basis by the updating of each attendance or visit, and be able to refer to other aspects of the patient's background which may be important, e.g. occupation and social history.

(4) Records can be used in such a way that patients are automatically recalled for important checks, such as repeat cervical smears, hypertensive therapy surveillance, and many other preventive and prophylactic procedures.

139

The following are methods of record-keeping in use at present.

Medical Record Envelope (FP5 and 6)

This envelope has had little modification since it was introduced in
1911. It is the property of the DHSS and is returned to the Family
Practitioner Committee after the patient's death. Its small size (7¼ in.
x 5 in.) is a major disadvantage. Writing tends to be cramped and
illegible, but, even more important, hospital letters and other records
rarely fit the envelope without being folded several times. The envelope
rapidly becomes bulky, and there is a tendency for doctors not to refer
to documents which have to be unfolded and then refolded.

A4 Folder

This record is based on paper of A4 size (11¾ x 8¼). First introduced
in two practices in Wantage (Hawkey *et al*., 1971; Loudon, 1975), a
record folder was designed which has a pocket on the inside of the front
of the folder, and a second pocket on the back. Record sheets of A4
size are attached by tags or soft metal strip to two spines which run
along the back of the folder. One major advantage of using a folder of
A4 size is that hospital reports and correspondence can be filed flat.
A second advantage is that the practitioner has more scope and space
to organise the record.

An A4 record, however, takes up one and a half times the space of
the present envelope. Curtis in 1974 surveyed 130 general practitioners
and found that 48 per cent would not have sufficient space to store A4
records.

So, although in 1973 the DHSS agreed in principle to the conversion
of general practice records to A4 (ECN 946 1973), little progress has
been made in view of the potential cost of the structural changes
which would be needed to store them. The secretarial cost of transfer-
ring the traditional record to A4 has been calculated as occupying one
secretary up to two years to transfer the records of one principal.
Finally, the problem of adapting an A4 record to one of traditional
size when a patient moves from one practice to another has been
encountered. The introduction of A4 records has understandably been
slow.

Family Folder

Another system is that in which all records of one family are stored together. They are made available whenever one member presents himself or herself. This has some advantages in practices where patients frequently see different doctors, but is probably not justified in other practices as a family record may rapidly become very bulky.

Problem Orientated Medical Record (POMR)

This type of record is known as 'problem orientated' because the whole record is based on the problems which patients have. It was originally introduced by Lawrence Weed in 1969 in the USA for hospital records. There are three basic components:

(1) The problem list.
(2) Background information package.
(3) Plan and progress notes.

1. The Problem List

When a patient first attends his problems are identified and numbered, for example:

(1) Acute Bronchitis.
(2) Rheumatoid Arthritis.
(3) Poor Housing.

All information in a POMR is entered, stored, retrieved, and used according to the problem to which it refers. When a problem has been resolved this is indicated on the problem list and ceases to be an active problem. For example, P3 — rehoused — satisfactory.

The doctor only needs to deal with the problems presented to him on any one occasion by the patient. If there is no new information on other problems these are left unchanged. The advantage of a problem list organised in this way is that the system reminds the doctor of the unresolved problems at each consultation.

2. The Background Information Package

This information again is usually obtained when the patient joins the practice list, although some doctors advise collecting it gradually. It has two components, the fixed and the changing information.

   (a) The fixed information – this consists of:
   Sex
   Date of Birth
   Previous Illnesses
   Immunisation
   Family History if relevant
   (b) The changing information – this consists of:
   Marital Status
   Occupation
   Address
   Screening Tests, e.g. Cervical Smear

This package is recorded separately and will obviously not need to be referred to on all occasions.

Some confusion arises between the phrases 'background information package' and 'data base'. The phrase 'data base' was originally used by Weed in its hospital context to include all the information in the 'background information package' *plus* the results of clinical examinations and laboratory tests.

3. The Plan and Progress Notes: SOAP

The progress notes are written for each current episode of attendance and only differ from normal record entries in being structured. The patient's complaint is dealt with under the headings:

   (a) *Subjective* – the patient's observations and complaints.
   (b) *Objective* – the results of examinations and investigations.
   (c) *Analysis* – a concise statement of the situation as the doctor sees it.
   (d) *Plan* – this consists of four components:
      (1)   The goal (or aim): to try and write down a realistic possible achievement, e.g. to get the diastolic BP below 100 in six weeks.
      (2)   Information required, e.g. the health visitor to check on accommodation.
      (3)   Action – whether and what prescription was given, certificates, etc.
      (4)   Patient education – note, verbatim if possible, what the patient has been told about his condition.

The advantages of writing the current entry in this way are that the doctor is obliged to structure his activities and actions logically. If another doctor sees the patient it is immediately apparent what plans the previous doctor had for action.

Secondary Uses for POMR

(1) Quality control of patient care. There is a record of the doctor's thoughts and decisions. Later these can be compared against outcome by the doctor himself to modify his future action.

(2) Education. If a medical student or trainee records in the SOAP pattern it is much easier to follow the logic (or absence of logic) of his actions. It is therefore a valuable teaching tool.

(3) Preventive medicine. The construction of the background information package enables one to see risk factors for the patient, such as incompleted immunisation schedules.

(4) Research. For a researcher doing a retrospective study of records the information is structured and readily identifiable.

Order out of Chaos

In many practices, even in training practices, the patient record is chaotic. When a patient is seen by a doctor other than his own (partners, locums, trainees) the 'record' may consist of well-nigh illegible jottings with sheets and hospital letters all jumbled up together. To enter information in a problem-orientated way is one method of structuring the record so that salient facts are more easily found. But there are other simpler methods of bringing order out of chaos, some of which can be carried out by the office staff, others which need the doctors' attention.

1. Notes Arranged in Chronological Order

It is a relatively simple task to arrange the record cards in order. Stapling and cellotape, popular in the past, have in many practices given way to punching a hole and using Treasury tags. With this method inserts or summary cards can be added with little effort. One of the advantages of carrying out this exercise is that the point where the previous record ended will be obvious to anyone making a fresh note, which helps to eliminate all the partly filled EC7s which fatten most record envelopes.

2. Letters and Reports Arranged in Order

Again it is a fairly simple task to arrange these in chronological order.
Problems arise with selection. Some doctors hoard every scrap of
information in case some test or nuance in a letter which is not
relevant at the time *might* be relevant later. Others are more brutal
and abstract without misgiving. If this task is delegated to office staff
it is important that the views of each individual doctor are known and
respected for the records of his patients.

3. Colour Codes on Record Envelopes

The Royal College of General Practitioners has agreed a colour code
for certain diseases, for example, black for an attempted suicide,
yellow for epilepsy, blue for hypertension. Patients with significant
conditions such as those indicated can be readily identified by a
colour tag on their envelopes to alert the doctor when they are seen.

The same system of record tagging can be used for any other condition or situation which the doctor may wish to identify. The RCGP
study on an Attitudes to Pregnancy Survey, for example, requires a
tag with APS to be fixed to the outside of the record envelope. In large
practices dealing with 15,000-30,000 patients it may be administrat-
ively easier to identify each doctor's patients by giving each doctor a
colour code and the displayed edge of the record carries this colour.
Alternatively each alphabetical shelf may have a different colour so
that misplaced records can be easily identified.

4. Emphasising Important Facts

Much of the written record is of a descriptive or provisional nature.
There are, however, in all records certain diagnoses or procedures
which are potentially relevant to any future consultation as an *aide-
mémoire* or classifier. Colour coding the envelope has limited possibilities. If important facts are underlined, boxed or starred on the
record itself, then they are less likely to be overlooked.

5. Summary Cards

A logical extension of boxing or underlining important facts on the
record is for these facts to be gathered together on a summary card.
Priority details might include diagnoses, operations, drug sensitivities.

Summary cards which the doctor can adapt for his own use can be obtained from the Family Practitioner Service. Maycock and colleagues have described a comprehensive system based on over-printing. Tait has described a system using specially printed cards. Summary cards can also be obtained from the Royal College of General Practitioners.

Repeat prescription cards are an example of a summary card being used regularly for management. These cards, in addition to the name and address of doctor and patient, state the drug, the dose, the frequency of administration, the quantity to be dispensed – all the information needed to make out a prescription. In addition the dates on which the drugs have been prescribed and the number of times the prescription can be repeated without the patient seeing the doctor should be entered. In many practices it is understood by patients that a prescription will not be repeated unless the card is presented.

The extensive use, and the potential misuse, of these cards has given rise to some disquiet but there is no doubt that they have proved a useful aid in practice management. It is important that the partners should review the system regularly to ensure that the proper safeguards are being observed.

Advantages and Uses of Structured Records

Having described the various types of manual record and some of the ways in which order can be imposed upon chaos, it is possible to look in more detail at the ways in which such records may be used.

(1) As an aid to better patient care. The ready availability of important facts, of past history with priority details, must result in diminished doctor frustration with greater efficiency in diagnosis and therapy.

(2) For increasing practice income. The presence of structured records encourages the use of an efficient call and recall system for procedures which attract item-of-service payments. Immunisations and cervical smears will be more efficiently organised if there is a system based on a structured record and an age-sex register. For those doctors who provide contraceptive services a system based on similar lines will encourage both this aspect of preventive medicine and higher practice income.

(3) For patient monitoring. The call and recall procedures described for preventive medicine can be extended into other aspects of care.

The tagged records of patients with diseases which need long-term regular supervision, such as hypertension and diabetes, can be used as the basis of a system of call and recall for regular surveillance. Structured records are in widespread use for antenatal care. Similar structuring for developmental examinations in children or for functional assessments of the elderly have clear advantages.

(4) Teaching. In a teaching practice one important function of the record is that it should be intelligible and useful to both partners and trainee. The use of records for teaching may be severely limited if it is not possible easily to extract relevant facts. How can a trainee, for example, be encouraged to believe regular long-term follow-up of diabetic patients is desirable if those patients who are diabetic cannot be identified?

(5) For research. Without structured records any form of epidemiological research in general practice is very difficult. Extraction of information from the record is frustrating and time-consuming. The use of summary cards makes collection of data easier. In some practices the use of summary cards has been extended into the maintenance of consultation recording systems and disease index registers (E book). Eimerl & Laidlaw, Pinsent and Howie have described the possibilities in detail.

The setting up and maintenance of an age-sex register, which can be regarded as a form of structured practice record, is increasingly being regarded not only as a research tool but as an important ingredient in good practice management. Comprehensive immunisation programmes, screening programmes for all ages, programmes to check the accuracy of capitation fee payments, all depend on an up-to-date age-sex register.

(6) For audit. The original meaning of the word audit is that of counting, measuring. The second stage is to interpret and analyse the results. Later the practitioner may wish to compare what is happening in his practice with what he thought was happening—or to compare what happens in his practice with what happens in other practices. But the first stage in audit is counting and without structured records, whether they be clinical or management records, counting is impossible. When looking at an appointment system, for example, discrepancies between time booked and time seen and a record of how long it takes a patient to see a doctor enables the practice to audit the efficiency of their system. Structured records facilitate the audit of many other aspects of practice. This matter is further discussed in Chapter 13.

Computers

This chapter has thus far considered manual records. We have no doubt, however, that an office revolution is beginning based on the silicon chip. Word processors are moving into larger businesses replacing the typewriter. An increasing number of general practitioners are dabbling with small computers in their practices. The General Medical Services Committee has commissioned a review by a computer consultancy. The RCGP Computer Working Party has published a report. Computer projects in Exeter and Oxford have proved their practicality and usefulness over a period of years.

It is not part of the remit of this book to talk about future possibilities. We have concentrated on guidelines for running a practice today. But, as we are convinced that the use of computers has the potential to change the way in which family medicine is practised, we believe that it is not too early to discuss the prospects.

What are the characteristics of computers which lead us to this view? The function of a computer is to accept information (which can be stored on discs or other forms of 'memory'), to manipulate it, juggle it, reproduce it, and to provide as output information in the form that is needed. The particular way in which stored information is manipulated (processed) at any one time depends on the programme which is plugged into the machine.

How is this relevant to general practice and how might computers be used? This question may be considered under five headings:

(1) As an aid to practice organisation. At a simple level, if the names, ages and addresses of the patients registered with the practice are entered into the computer memory, other facts can also be entered for each patient: immunisation state, date of last cervical smear, date of acceptance on the practice list, date of acceptance for contraceptive services; with suitable programmes the computer could produce lists of eleven-year-old girls who have not had rubella immunisation, of patients whose FP1001 is due the following month. With a suitable machine, sticky labels can be printed enabling reminders to be sent.

A second example would be the printing of repeat prescriptions. If the information normally recorded on the repeat prescription card is entered into the computer memory and numbered, when the appropriate programme is operating the receptionist types in the required number. The printer attached to the computer then prints out the prescription with name, address of patient, type, quantity and administrative details of drug, name and address of doctor, together with the number of repeats still available before the patient sees the doctor.

Similar organisation programmes and packages can be envisaged for financial analysis, for administration and for appointment systems.

(2) As a clinical aid. We stress elsewhere that we believe practice organisation directly affects clinical care. As more of the patient record is entered into computer memory the possible uses of the computer become more overtly clinical. Its use as an aid in surveillance of chronic disease is a direct extension of call and recall for immunisation schemes. Programmes exist which warn of drug sensitivities or incompatibilities when diagnoses and drug therapy are entered. The practitioner could start analysing his own prescribing patterns, the effects of long-term treatment on chronic disease could correlate drug side-effects in different age groups. The implications for self-audit and for research are enormous.

(3) As a diagnostic aid. The use of a computer to recognise abnormal ECG patterns has already been described by Hoyle. Dove has described his use of a computer for patient history-taking. A programme has recently been demonstrated in which a patient with a headache 'talks' to a computer and the computer produces a diagnosis with the degree of probability of the diagnosis being correct at the end of the interrogation. The use of computers in this way, as a machine which might be interposed between patient and doctor, has implications for family medicine which will certainly be a hot controversial topic during the next decade.

(4) As a source of information. Information from any source can be stored in a computer—the quantity stored depending on the size of the computer's memory. It is possible to envisage drug information, the Red Book, clinical information from medical textbooks, being stored with programmes to extract those parts needed by a particular practice. Programmes have already been devised which instruct as to the immunisation requirements for travellers to different countries, sources of vaccine, and contra-indications to immunisation. The attached printer then prints out the necessary documents (prescription, claim forms, certificates, bills).

The probability is that instead of storing such information on practice computers (which would require a very large memory) use will be made of data banks, such as Prestel, with individual practices hooking into the section they need.

(5) As a means of communication. If practice computers or terminals

can communicate with data banks, it is probable that before long ways will be devised for different computers and different makes of computer to communicate with each other without printed paper being issued by one computer and put into another. This would open a new world of communication – between practice and practice, practice and FPC, practice and hospital. The availability of transmitted information to unauthorised people can be limited in a number of ways, including passwords and 'closed-user groups'. It is possible to imagine the DHSS transmitting alterations to the Red Book (SFAs) directly to practice computers, or the Committee on Safety of Drugs issuing warnings concerning a particular drug in a similar way through a closed-user group which consisted of all general-practitioner principals.

As can be judged from the above, we believe that the use of computers in general practice will affect not only the way records are kept or the way the practice is organised, but will alter the whole scale of magnitude of the information available to the general practitioner in his own practice. There will be repercussions on audit, on education, on research, on the expectations of patients and doctors and eventually on the whole future of general practice itself.

References and Further Reading

Dawes, K.S. 'Survey of General Practitioner Records', *British Medical Journal*, 3 (1972), pp. 219-23.

Eimerl, T.S. & Laidlaw, A.S. *A Handbook for Research in General Practice*, 2nd edition (Edinburgh and London: E. & S. Livingstone, 1969).

Elliot, A., Valdez, N., Dempsey, C. & Cooper, P. 'An Evaluation of the A4 Folder System in General Practice', *Journal of the Royal College of General Practitioners*, 29 (1979), pp. 85-9.

Hawkey, J.K., Loudon, I.S.L., Greenhalgh, G.P. & Bungay, G.T. 'New Record Folder for Use in General Practice', *British Medical Journal*, 4 (1971), pp. 667-70.

Howie, J.G.R. *Research in General Practice* (London: Croom Helm, 1979).

Loudon, I.S.L. 'Record-Keeping in General Practice', *Update*, 10 (1975), pp. 259-67.

Maycock, C. 'G.P. records: Paediatric Development Card', *British Medical Journal*, 2 (1979), pp. 1453-4.

Pinsent, R.F.J.H. 'The Evolving Age-Sex Register', *Journal of the Royal College of General Practitioners*, 16 (1968), pp. 127-34.

Tait, I.G. 'The Clinical Record in British General Practice', *British Medical Journal*, 2 (1977), pp. 683-8.

Weed, L. *Medical Records, Medical Education and Patient Care* (Cleveland Press of Case Western Reserve University, 1969).

Zander, L., Beresford, S.A.A. & Thomas, P. 'Medical Records in General Practice', *Occasional Paper 5: Journal of the Royal College of General Practitioners* (1978).

Of the adjectives applied to general practitioners the word 'busy' is one of the most common. Many patients and many doctors visualise general practitioners as being almost under siege, confronted with a vast number of patients constantly and simultaneously wanting to see them, and living in a precarious state of balance in which the doctor's supply of time barely meets the demands made upon it.

There are good historical reasons for this image. The most obvious is that with the introduction of the National Health Service in 1948 it was accepted in a Western society for the first time that open access to general medical care should be available for the whole population of a country on a continuing basis day and night throughout the year. Certainly at that time doctors were fearful that, given a completely free service without any direct financial involvement by the patient, they would face impossible demands and might not be able to meet all the requests that they received.

Furthermore, at that time a large number of general practitioners were practising single-handed. By today's standards their administrative support was rudimentary. Most did not have a secretary or a reception-ist, and many relied on their wives and families for help.

It is hardly surprising that the image of the 'busy' doctor arose although few general practitioners could define accurately the amount of work they were doing.

Recognition that unless a general practitioner can analyse what is going on within the practice he is unlikely to be able to make reasoned changes to improve its efficiency has been slow in gaining general acceptance.

Organisational Revolution

In the 1950s, pioneered largely by the Royal College of General Practitioners, a variety of aids to practice organisation were introduced. The employment of secretaries using typewriters and dictaphones was encouraged. A variety of new ways of organising and abstracting records was introduced, of which age-sex registers (introduced by the Birmingham Research Unit of the College) and the diagnostic register originally called the 'E' book (introduced by Dr T.S. Eimerl) were among the most important.

About the same time a growing number of general practitioners began to analyse their own work and to keep records of the number of consultations and home visits they were doing. The introduction of appointment systems helped them to analyse their own workload and provided a baseline for comparisons of the amount, type and range of work carried out.

At first it was mainly the enthusiasts and research workers in general practice, a tiny minority of general practitioners as a whole, who were most interested. However, as time went on and reports such as the *Present State and Future Needs* of the Royal College of General Practitioners appeared, more general practitioners found it interesting to be able to compare their workload with that of their colleagues and to learn about new ideas of organisation from them. A study of the journals of general practice in the 1950s shows a large number of articles reporting appointment systems and workload studies in different type of practices.

During the 1960s and 1970s these ideas spread. They ceased to be the prerogative of a small minority but became common practice of first hundreds and then thousands of general practitioners. Nowadays, indeed, it is expected that all training practices will have age-sex registers and will be able to demonstrate their use to the vocational trainees (*Journal of the Royal College of General Practitioners*, 1977). Similarly, the number of practices which are able to analyse consultations by diagnosis and which have lists of patients with various chronically handicapping conditions is growing all the time.

Since all these systems cost both time and money and involve general practitioners in additional work the questions are bound to be asked, 'What is their purpose? What is their value? How can they help me in running my practice?'

Advantages

The advantages to general practitioners of knowing what is going on in their practices can be considered under four main headings:

(1) Practice management and planning
(2) Clinical standards
(3) Improving income

(4) Professional morale

1. Practice Management

General practitioners have to take decisions about a whole variety of problems, both clinical and management. All general practitioners are daily brought into contact with clinical problems but until recently the nature of management problems and the influence they had on clinical matters were largely unrecognised.

General practitioners have to take decisions about the number of staff to employ, their qualifications, their duties, and the degree of responsibility which can appropriately be delegated to them. They have to decide whether or not to have an appointment system. If there is an appointment system how many patients should be booked each hour? They have to decide whether or not their appointment system is working satisfactorily.

There are three considerations which in our view make the gathering of management information and feedback essential:

(a) Decision-taking should be based on fact.

It is obvious that the ability to take such decisions must depend upon the information available to the decision-maker. Yet paradoxically, because of its history, general practice has grown up in a tradition of decision-taking by hunch, often without the benefit of (and sometimes in the face of) facts.

Almost all studies of decision-taking in industrial organisations emphasise the importance of rational thinking in the light of fact. One of the main advantages of regular documentation of various practice activities such as the number of consultations, and the number of patients seen by each doctor, is that the general practitioner partners who, as was shown in Chapter 7, are the apex of the decision-taking process, are better informed and therefore likely to take better decisions. Put another way, without some form of feedback about what is actually happening decisions about systems and staff are taken in the dark.

(b) Basic statistics are necessary for comparison.

An allied and important consideration is that once basic statistics about a practice have been established, such as the total number of patients on the lists, their age-sex distribution, and rate of contact with the doctor, it becomes possible to compare the practice with other practices both nationally and regionally. Substantial variation from colleagues is an indication for review which may in itself lead to new ways of solving problems.

(c) Basic statistics can show trends.

Finally, knowing that information is being collected and being able to see it and discuss it over a period of time helps the practice staff morale considerably. It may enable partners to adjust staffing or systems long before outright complaints and grievances occur. For example, in one of our practices a steadily rising quantity of work in the treatment room was shown in the quarterly and annual returns. A decision was therefore taken to increase the number of nursing hours in the practice before grievance arose with the practice nurses.

Vital Statistics

One group of figures is so important that we regard them as 'vital statistics'. We recommend that they should be kept by every general practitioner who works a personal list system and by every group of doctors who do not.

The number of times each patient comes to the surgery on average during the year is known as the *annual consultation rate* and the average number of times each patient is visited at home each year is the *home visiting rate*. The two added together form the total *doctor-patient contact rate*.

If a record is kept of the number of consultations by each doctor's registered patients (or all consultations for a group) and the number of home visits then these three figures can be calculated quite easily. Big changes can occur within a few years. It is only by looking at these statistics that practitioners can define trends so that they may have facts on which to adjust their practice policies.

Example 1: Practice Policies. The following figures were kept for the six consecutive years 1974 to 1979 for the patients registered with one of the authors in a three-partner practice in Exeter. The general trend of both the consultation rate and the home visiting rate (and of the total doctor-patient contact rate) is downwards. Furthermore, they show a fall in the home visiting rate per patient of as much as a third in six years.

Table 13.1: Vital Statistics

Year	Surgery consultation rate per patient per year	Home visiting rate per patient per year	Total doctor-patient contact rate per year
1974	2.85	0.50	3.35
1975	2.79	0.43	3.23
1976	2.65	0.35	2.99
1977	2.46	0.36	2.82
1978	2.68	0.41	3.09
1979	2.56	0.33	2.89

In this practice over the years in question two policy decisions had been taken by the partners both of which might have caused an increase in the doctor-patient contact rate. In the first place, a policy of encouraging preventive procedures within the practice was increasingly and systematically pursued. In the second, a move was made towards increasing explanation to the patient while reducing the number of prescriptions issued.

In practice it could be demonstrated that neither of these policies had resulted in an increased patient-doctor contact rate. They were therefore continued.

Example 2: Personal Care. When in one practice the partners changed their policy from letting patients see the first doctor available to guiding them to see their own doctor, the question naturally arose – was the policy working? Extraction from the figures showed that from April 1978 to March 1980 the percentage of patients who saw their own doctor rose from 48 at the beginning of the period to 68 at the end. Receptionists as well as doctors found these facts interesting. The measures which had been instituted were judged to be working successfully, and a joint decision was taken to continue.

In the hurly-burly of the day-to-day flow of patients going through a reception desk it is often not possible for the staff to see such broad general trends, and feedback of this kind greatly adds to the interest of their job.

2. Clinical Standards

It is increasingly being recognised that clinical standards depend on record-keeping (*Journal of the Royal College of General Practitioners*, 1980). It is difficult for a doctor systematically to organise care for a patient if he has no management plan. The care of a hypertensive patient, for example, depends on blood-pressure readings being recorded at regular intervals. Similarly, the care of patients with asthma increasingly depends on good documentation of serial peak-flow readings. Care of patients with epilepsy depends on a record of fits and effects of treatment. We are all human and without notes we cannot always remember what target result or plan of campaign was agreed with the patient.

If a recorded management plan is necessary for the patient's own doctor it is even more necessary for partners and colleagues in these days of group practice, vocational training, longer holidays and rotas.

One of the great advantages of miniaturisation (Gray, 1978) is that monitoring systems for the chronically handicapped are increasingly coming within the power of general practitioners to control and use. Within the last few years, for example, mini peak-flow meters and portable machines for testing blood sugars have become available at prices most general practices can afford. Thus it becomes possible to monitor asthmatics and diabetics as accurately now as most hospital clinics could do only a few years ago. In this way standards of care can rise quickly and the science of medicine be made available to a much greater number of patients in the population.

Furthermore, once there are good record systems it becomes possible to know what is going on in a whole group of patients with a common condition. Diagnostic registers, for example, make it possible for a general practitioner to identify all his patients with asthma, diabetes, epilepsy or hypertension, and examine the effectiveness of his care.

Such analysis of the clinical record is increasingly being carried out in training practices both by trainers and trainees. The first results are sobering (Kratky, 1977). It is only by examining what we are trying to do and whether we are succeeding that standards can eventually be improved.

3. Improving Income

General practitioners are independent contractors (Chapter 2). A proportion of their income depends on item-of-service fees for preventive medicine. In Britain the average income of general practitioners from these fees is only about 7 per cent of the total NHS income (Chapter 8), whereas in some of the authors' practices much higher fees are currently being obtained.

For example, in one of our practices with three partners, a total list size of 6,639 patients, and an age-sex structure approximating to the national average, the item-of-service fees for the quarter ending 31 March 1980 were as follows:

	£	Annual equivalent (£)
Maternity medical services	711	2,844
Contraceptive care	656	2,624
Immunisations	624	2,496
Cervical cytology tests	197	788
Night visits	101	404
Emergency treatment	27	108
Dental haemorrhage	0	0
	£2,316	£9,264 p.a.

In this practice the total percentage of item-of-service fees as a proportion of NHS practice income at 31 March 1980 was 17.6 per cent. On analysing why this practice can have two and a half times the amount of income from item-of-service fees as the national average, it appears that the income depends on the systems which were set up to enable the partners to know what was going on in the practice.

Example 3: Cervical Cytology. In the quarter ending March 1978 the partners reviewed the current regulations governing NHS payments for cervical cytology (Red Book, Statement of Fees and Allowances, para. 28.1). It immediately became clear that some of the partners were not familiar with the regulations and on relatively few occasions were claiming the appropriate fee on Form FP74. There was unanimous agreement to start increasing the practice income from this source with the results shown in Table 13.2. These figures show a fourfold increase in practice income for cervical cytology over the two-year period. In other words, the practice income from cervical cytology fees rose from a rate of £193 a year to a rate of £789 a year within two years.

Example 4: Tetanus Immunisation. The partners in the same practice read with concern about the death from tetanus of a fit middle-aged man in the United Kingdom in 1979. A sample of the medical records showed that in relatively few cases was the tetanus immunisation status of its adult patients recorded although the proportion of children immunised was high.

Table 13.2: Cervical Cytology

Date 1978	Quarterly payments for cervical cytology	
31.3.1978	£48.30	Cytology campaign started
30.6.1978	£66.70	
30.9.1978	£62.70	
31.12.1978	£84.10	
1979		
31.3.1979	£72.50	
30.6.1979	£104.40	
30.9.1979	£159.80	
31.12.1979	£102.00	
1980		
31.3.1980	£197.20	

The three partners decided to initiate a tetanus preventive campaign by offering patients a tetanus immunisation from the practice nurse when they consulted for other conditions.

The increase in workload for the practice sisters in the treatment was immediate (Appendix C) and the figures for the quarter ending 31 March 1980 showed that the sisters immunised 180 adults during the quarter (an annual rate if maintained of about one in eight of all the adult patients). The consequences for the practice income have been considerable as shown in Table 13.3.

Table 13.3: Increased NHS Income after Tetanus Immunisation Campaign

Quarter ending	Practice income shown in NHS quarterly returns from Family Practitioner Committee	
30 June 1978	£310)	
30 September 1978	£274)	Income for four
31 December 1978	£324)	successive quarters 1978/79
31 March 1979	£336)	= £1,244
Tetanus immunisation campaign started		
30 June 1979	£444)	
30 September 1979	£609)	Income for four
31 December 1979	£543)	successive quarters 1979/80
31 March 1980	£623)	= £2,219

The World Health Organisation advocates that primary care is the natural setting for practical preventive medicine for patients in their local communities. The primary health care team, working together closely in general practice, is ideally equipped to bring practical preventive medicine to the vast mass of the population. In the United Kingdom the National Health Service appropriately recognises this responsibility and has provided several financial incentives to undertake it.

That such preventive medicine should be undertaken in general practice is desirable for patients, good for the health of the community and is in the professional interests of the general practitioner and his nursing colleagues who gain in professional satisfaction. Moreover, the practice gains financially.

4. Morale

One of the most important touchstones in determining a doctor's attitude to general practice lies in his attitude to the job itself. In Britain today there are doctors who find general practice tedious, boring, and exasperating, who are out of sympathy with the demands of their patients and see themselves as harried and harassed in their everyday work. Such doctors have low professional morale, and may be heard complaining about their patients, their terms of service and the large amount of trivia in their work.

Side by side with these doctors, sometimes even in the same street, are general practitioners who find general practice intellectually demanding, professionally stimulating and emotionally satisfying. They like their job, are ready and willing to accept the new responsibilities, and are prepared to spend substantial amounts of their free time researching, teaching, or developing their discipline.

It was Irvine in 1978 who first identified these two populations of doctors but subsequently Robinson (1979), a former Chairman of the Patients Association, also commented on them. 'Good practices are getting better so fast that they are almost beyond criticism . . . By contrast the rump of the profession, often working in areas with highest morbidity and mortality, looks worse and worse.'

We believe that one of the main differences between these two groups of doctors is that the one accepts life as it comes, and in the absence of information and feedback has no way of making logical changes in the way he organises his practice, whereas the other knows what is going on and can do something logical and practical if things are going wrong. Moreover, in the second group positive encouragement is given to both staff and partners if feedback shows that the practice is working well and that practice policies are proving successful.

The doctor no longer feels a helpless prisoner of forces beyond his or her control. It is our experience that once practices do organise feedback and do know what is going on then professional morale rises dramatically. We have no doubt that information systems, whether they are in organisational, clinical or financial terms are to the benefit of patients, doctors and staff.

To have reached this point in a chapter on audit without having mentioned the word must constitute some sort of record. Audit involves counting and measuring, followed by analysis. This is what this chapter has been all about.

References

Gray, D.J. Pereira. 'General Practitioners and the Independent Contractor Status', *Journal of the Royal College of General Practitioners*, 27 (1977), pp. 750-6.
———— James Mackenzie Lecture 1977. 'Feeling at Home', *Journal of the Royal College of General Practitioners*, 28 (1978), pp. 6-17.
———— 'The Key to Personal Care', *Journal of the Royal College of General Practitioners*, 29 (1979), pp. 666-78.
Irvine, D.H. 'The Future of the College', *Journal of the Royal College of General Practitioners*, 28 (1978), pp. 146-53.
Journal of the Royal College of General Practitioners. Editorial, Age-sex Registers, 27 (1977), pp. 515-17.
———— Editorial, Systematic Surveillance, 30 (1980), p. 2.
Kratky, A.P. 'An Audit of the Care of Diabetics in One General Practice', *Journal of the Royal College of General Practitioners*, 27 (1977), pp. 536-43.
National Health Service (Family Practitioner Services), *Statement of Fees and Allowances Payable to General Medical Practitioners, The Red Book* (London: DHSS, n.d.)
Robinson, J. *The Lancet*, 2 (1979), p. 211.
Royal College of General Practitioners. *Present State and Future Needs of General Practice.* Reports from General Practice No. 16 (London: *Journal of the Royal College of General Practitioners*, 1973 and 1976).

PART SIX: THE WIDER WORLD

14 INTERESTS OUTSIDE THE PRACTICE

The family doctor, like other professional people, will almost certainly become involved with interests outside his practice. Some of these will be an inevitable consequence of his being a general practitioner, such as being eligible to vote for his representative on the Local Medical Committee (LMC), whilst others may be an expected duty of the 'village doctor', such as presidency of the village Cricket Club.

In this chapter we shall look at outside interests which are directly related to being a medical practitioner. These have been divided into those which are likely to be done for love and those which are carried out for money.

For Love

The British Medical Association, the Royal College of General Practitioners and the Local Medical Committee are the three medical organisations with which general practitioners are most likely to be involved. They represent the general practitioners' interests in the field of medical politics, training, continuing education and research. All three have a local structure, which means that the general practitioner can seek advice or participate in the organisation at a local level. In the case of the British Medical Association, the local structure depends upon the local division. The Royal College of General Practitioners has faculties at a regional level administered by a Faculty Board. The Local Medical Committee operates over an area identical to that administered by the Family Practitioner Committee and, in some cases, even has district subdivisions so that individual general practitioners may refer to their local district committee of the LMC. The central body for Local Medical Committees is the General Medical Services Committee.

Although the Royal College of General Practitioners, the British Medical Association and the General Medical Services Committee have interests in common in the field of general practice, their functions are mainly complementary, and their membership is obtained in different ways.

163

The Local Medical Committee

All general practitioners in contract with a Family Practitioner Committee have a vote in electing their representative to serve on the Local Medical Committee. Thus, the LMC is the only truly representative body of all the general practitioners working in the National Health Service. At the local level, it is the responsibility of the LMC to watch over the interests of its members and to negotiate the settlement of local medical difficulties. It is also responsible for appointing the medical members of the Family Practitioner Committee and its sub-committees. It thus has considerable influence over medical administration in the general practitioner's area. In particular, it appoints members to the local Medical Practices Committee which itself appoints doctors to single-handed practices, to the Medical Services Committee which is responsible for investigating complaints made against family doctors, and to the Local Obstetric Committee which, amongst other things, is responsible for the appointment of general practitioners to the obstetric list. A typical LMC agenda is illustrated in Table 14.1. Elections to the Local Medical Committee are on a constituency basis. Each general practitioner has his own elected representative member. He is, therefore, able to raise individual problems directly with his own representative.

Each year each local medical committee sends a number of its members to represent it at the annual Conference of Local Medical Committees and each year several local medical committees together elect a member to serve on the General Medical Services Committee (GMSC). The GMSC is the executive of the conference of LMCs. It negotiates with the Department of Health and Social Security on the terms and conditions of service for general practitioners working within the National Health Service as the sole representative of all general practitioners. Members of the GMSC are not necessarily members of the BMA.

The LMCs are financed by statutory levy on every general practitioner in their area. In addition, there is a voluntary levy on general practitioners for activities not specified by statute and for the General Medical Services Defence Trust – the general practitioners' fighting fund.

The British Medical Association

The British Medical Association is a voluntary association with members in all branches of the medical profession, both in and out of the National Health Service. Its prime objectives, as stated in the Memorandum of Association, are 'to promote the medical and allied sciences, and to maintain the honour and interests of the medical profession'.

Table 14.1: Local Medical Committee Agenda

---

1. Apologies for absence.
2. Minutes of the previous meeting.
3. Matters arising from the minutes.
4. Report on the Annual Conference of Representatives of the LMCs.
5a. Election of member on FPC dispensing sub-committee.
5b. Election of a member on North Wessex Disablement Advisory Committee.
5c. Election of a member to the Ophthalmic Service Committee. (Deputies may be appointed for all these representatives.)
6. Appointment of practice nurses (see enclosed memorandum).
7. Storage of drugs in surgeries; to receive a memorandum from the police.
8. To receive reports from representatives of:
   a) The regional medical committee.
   b) The GMS committee.
   c) The Area Health Care Planning Team (mental illness).
9. To receive accounts for the year ended 31 March.
10. District sub-committee reports.
11. Matters arising from circulars received.
   a) GMSC circulars.
     i) Review Body report.
     ii) Cameron Fund Limited.
   b) DHSS circulars.
     i) Senior management education and training.
     ii) Prescription charges (revised forms FP57).
12. Mileage allowances for attendances at courses.
13. New forms FP19 (temporary residence).
14. Payments for loss or damage of oxygen equipment.
15. Trainees, allowance for additional car.
16. Remuneration of general medical practitioners (Review Body increases).
17. Any other business.
18. Date of next meeting.

Signed, Clerk to the Committee.

It is both a registered company, limited by guarantee, and an independent trade union listed under the Trade Union and Labour Relations Act 1974. Four of its standing committees representing the Hospital Medical Service, General Practice, Junior Hospital Doctors and Community Medicine are recognised by the Secretary of State for Social Service as sole negotiators with the Department of Health and Social Services on all matters relating to their respective branches of the profession.

In addition to its trade union function, the BMA has a range of committees to deal with specific aspects of medical practice. There is a Private Practice Committee which, among other things, negotiates fees for its members with non-NHS bodies including other government departments. There is an Ethical Committee which considers a very wide

range of matters from the use of torture in interrogation, and the
confidentiality of medical data, to disputes between individual members
of the profession. The Board of Science and Education provides an
authoritative professional response to many matters of public interest.
On behalf of the Association it brings together the views of all branches
of the profession on such matters as the age of consent, seat-belts and
abortions. It also advises on the library at BMA House, distributes
awards and prizes, and arranges the annual clinical meetings of the
association. There are many other committees such as those for the
Armed Forces, Occupational Health and Medical Charities. The
British Medical Journal is highly regarded world-wide and is free to
members.

At a local level, the division is a forum for members of all branches
of the profession and encourages interchange and understanding between
them in both the medical and political fields. The regional secretariat
provides a 'trouble-shooting' back-up to the shop-steward activities of
the Divisional Honorary Secretary. All divisions elect representatives
to the Annual Representative Meeting. In this way they have a voice
in the decision-making of the Association, as the Representative Body
is the policy-making body of the Association and the Council, its
executive, is bound by the decisions of the Representative Body. It
therefore behoves every general practitioner to be a member of the
Association in order to play his or her full part as a responsible member
of the medical profession.

The Royal College of General Practitioners

The Royal College of General Practitioners was founded as the College
of General Practitioners in 1952. Its membership has grown to nearly
9,000 and a high proportion of new entrants to general practice sit its
membership examination. Whilst the other two organisations concern
themselves with representation of doctors' interests in the political
field and the provision of supporting services the RCGP is primarily
concerned with raising the standard of general practice through education,
improvements in practice organisation, and by encouraging research.
Many members have played an active part in the larger research projects
of the College, one of the best known being the Oral Contraception
Study. The RCGP publishes a monthly journal of general practice, the
Journal of the Royal College of General Practitioners, and a growing
list of occasional papers relevant to general practice. Like the BMA
subscription the RCGP subscription is a tax-allowable practice expense.

The College is organised in regional faculties, each being administered by a Faculty Board. Members and associates are allotted to the faculty within whose area they reside, although they may elect to change to another faculty if it is more convenient. Most faculties hold regular meetings throughout their areas. Local education and research groups may be formed and most postgraduate centres have a College representative.

Because of its interest in medical education, the College is particularly active in all vocational training schemes. Where these are in operation the College tutor and the course organiser are usually to be found working together. The book *The Future General Practitioner, Learning and Teaching* (1972) was one of the first attempts to analyse and describe the content of general practice. Not surprisingly it is considered essential reading for all those interested in teaching general practice.

Other Organisations

In most areas of the country there are established local medical societies which play an active part in the professional life of the locality. Nowadays many of these hold their meetings in postgraduate medical centres. For a small subscription they usually provide an interesting medical and social programme. A local society often provides a doctor new to the area with a forum where he may meet colleagues in both general practice and hospital practice.

For Money

Medical earnings from all sources inside and outside the practice are usually paid into the common partnership pool. Hence the partners' agreement to the acceptance of outside appointments is essential. A clear agreement as to who gets the money must be made before the appointment is accepted. This should include agreement on superannuation and other benefits.

Clinical Work in Hospitals and Health Authority Clinics

There is increasing opportunity for doctors with special interests and skills to do sessional work in hospitals and health authority clinics. Most appointments are currently paid at the clinical assistant grade but new appointments should be made at the hospital practitioner grade which properly recognises special skill. Whilst such work inevitably takes the doctor away from his general practice patients, it often benefits his practice in that he is able to maintain a high standard of expertise in his chosen field, and this often benefits both his patients and his partners in the practice.

Care must be taken that pursuing an interest does not cost the partnership money. For example, the doctor may work in an Area Health Authority family planning clinic on a sessional basis and find that he does all the family planning work for patients of his practice at a relatively small fee; whereas if he had provided a practice family planning service, the total reimbursement under the FPC contraceptive service would have been much greater. On the other hand, work in child health clinics, whilst often reducing a practice's income from the immunisations, usually will result in a net financial gain to the partnership from the sessional payments.

Work in additional clinical fields provides useful and interesting contacts. It is this aspect rather than money earned which is the main attraction to many general practitioners. The doctor's primary commitment must be to his practice and patients. Such sessional work cannot in our opinion exceed more than five half-days without loss of continuity of patient care.

School Medical Officers

Many practices provide medical services for residential schools within the practice area. It is common for such schools to retain the services of a particular practitioner as the 'school doctor'. In that case, not only will he be responsible for the day-to-day health of the pupils and staff (who are usually registered on his 'medical list') but he will also be called upon to carry out a large number of duties outside the National Health Service. These are mostly in the field of preventive medicine and include the following:

(a) Advising the headmaster or governing body in matters of health.

(b) Liaison with house masters and reporting to them or to the school matron fitness for activities of individual pupils.

(c) Epidemiological control within the school.

(d) Reporting annually on the health of the school and the sanitary condition of the premises. It is usual for the medical officer to be available to inspect drainage, sanitary provision, the dormitories, studies and common-rooms, lighting, cleanliness and heating of classrooms; also water, milk, and food supplies and kitchen hygiene.

(e) The administration of the sanatorium and direction of nursing staff duties.

(f) Admission examinations of pupils, periodic medical examinations and examinations when a pupil leaves the school.

(g) The proper keeping of medical records and regulations.

(h) The control of disinfection and hygienic disposal of refuse.

(i) Reports to parents or guardians.

(j) Medical examinations for the services, universities, employment medical advisory service, sub aqua clubs, etc.

(k) Correspondence with university medical officers.

These duties command a special fee, usually paid termly. Special surgeries are commonly held at the school for the convenience of staff and pupils.

The Medical Officers of Schools Association is an organisation which represents doctors working with schools. It arranges national meetings about topics of interest to school doctors. It also publishes the *Handbook of School Health* (15th edition, 1975), a very useful guide for school doctors and all others who are concerned in the health and welfare of young people. The Association also publishes regular news letters.

From time to time, the Medical Officers of Schools Association and the BMA publish a recommended scale of fees for school medical officers. It must be emphasised that no fee can be claimed for any duty which is covered by the National Health Service Act 1946, but fees are due for the additional duties outlined above. In 1978 the Price Commission approved a recommended fee of £7.50 per pupil per year. It should be noted that the Association of Governing Bodies of Public Schools has advised that 'all schools should from time to time review the fees payable to part-time medical officers to ensure that they are properly remunerated'. Since no two schools are identical, the scale referred to above should be taken as a guide for negotiating the appropriate fee in each individual case.

Other Appointments

In any area, the scope for additional appointments for doctors is considerable. Doctors who work on a part-time basis to service the needs of various government departments are usually termed Treasury Medical Officers. They may advise government departments on the fitness of prospective employees, the prognosis in staff who are sick, and on whether or not staff should be retired prematurely on health grounds. Main regional centres require police surgeons, and factories large and small are required by the Factory Act to have a named medical adviser.

Fees for all such appointments are negotiated and recommended by the Private Practice Committee of the BMA. However, doctors are always advised to negotiate an appropriate fee in the light of the expected work. For example, a small factory producing heavy industrial products may require a good deal more time than a larger light industrial concern.

Teaching

Many doctors enjoy teaching. Opportunities now exist in general practice for taking part in the undergraduate teaching programmes of most medical schools, in training future general practitioners through vocational training schemes, and by acting as a general practitioner trainer. A few doctors become course organisers and even fewer work part-time in direct association with the university departments of general practice.

Although those who take part generally do so from sheer enthusiasm, increased income can result from these activities. Medical schools pay an honorarium to the general practitioner supervisors, while general practitioner trainers receive the trainer's grant at the rate of £2,550 a year (1980) for the time a trainee is placed with them. The recommendation of the Joint Committee on Postgraduate Training for General Practice is that trainers should set aside at least two sessions per week for teaching their trainee and in addition should participate regularly in the local trainers' workshop. Course organisers are paid the same sum annually as general practitioner trainers, but do not have a trainee attached to them in their practices. Doctors teaching at vocational training or other postgraduate courses are entitled to a lecture fee for each session given. All this represents a considerable change from the situation which existed only a very few years ago. It reflects the importance now attached to training for general practice.

References and Further Reading

Handbook of School Health. Issued by Medical Officers of Schools Association, 15th edition (London: H.K. Lewis and Co. Ltd, 1975).
History of the British Medical Association 1832-1932. Compiled by E.M. Little (London: BMA, 1932).
Journal of the Royal College of General Practitioners, 27 (1977), no. 184. This is the 'Silver Jubilee number' and commemorates the 25th anniversary of the founding of the (then) College of General Practitioners on 19 November 1952.
Vaughan, P. *Doctors' Commons* (London: Heinemann, 1959).

15 THE SETTING: THE PRACTICE WITHIN THE HEALTH SERVICE

Diversity within a small area is a characteristic of Britain. Visitors used to the Rockies, the Plains or the Veldt are surprised how quickly they pass from town to country, to isolated communities, and back again. General practice reflects this diversity. Within fifty miles of any city the whole range of different types of practice can be found: the large group practice, the small practice, the one-man practice; the urban practice where all the patients may live within a half-mile radius, the rural practice where the practice area is commonly one hundred square miles or more; practices in health centres, in adapted or purpose-built premises, branch surgeries in the back room of the village shop. Each type of practice, each location, has its own particular problems and its own compensations.

There is, however, one factor common to all. Each general practitioner in the National Health Service has a contract with the Department of Health and Social Security. In England and Wales the contract states that he will practise according to Schedule 1 of the NHS Regulations 1974. In Scotland and in Northern Ireland the position is different. The differences involve not only the contract but also the organisation of the NHS in Scotland and Northern Ireland. The main differences are outlined in Appendices I and J.

NHS Regulations 1974

These regulations consist of nine parts and three schedules. The nine parts define the responsibilities of Family Practitioner Committees. The first of the three schedules lays down the terms of service for general practitioners. The duties of a general practitioner to the patients on his general medical list are summarised in paragraph 13:

a doctor shall render to his patients all necessary and appropriate personal medical services of the type usually provided by general medical practitioners. He shall do so at his practice premises or, if the condition of his patient so requires, elsewhere in his practice area. Such services include arrangements for referring patients as

171

necessary to the hospital and specialist services, the general ophthalmic services, and advice to enable them to take advantage of the local authority services. Except in an emergency this paragraph shall not impose an obligation on the doctor to provide maternity medical service unless he has undertaken to do so.

Organisation of the National Health Service

The way in which the National Health Service has been run in England and Wales since April 1974 was laid down in 1972 in a publication from the DHSS called *Management Arrangements for the Reorganised National Health Service.* The framework of the organisation, as quoted from this publication, was planned as follows:

(a) There are to be *Area* Health Authorities (AHA)—including some Area Health Authorities (Teaching) (AHA(T)) with particular medical and dental teaching responsibilities, accountable to *Regional* Health Authorities (RHA), who are in turn accountable to the *Secretary of State* for the effectiveness and efficiency of the services provided.

(b) These AHAs are to be coterminous geographically with the new local authorities (counties and metropolitan districts) which are to be set up outside London, and with the present London Boroughs or combinations of London Boroughs.

(c) Each AHA is to be required by statute to set up a *Family Practitioner Committee* (FPC) to administer the contracts of practitioners.

(d) There is to be statutory provision for the recognition of *professional advisory machinery*, from which RHAs, AHAs and FPCs will draw advice.

(e) *Community Health Councils* (CHC) are to be established to represent the views of the public to the AHAs.

The paper went on to lay down the administrative structure at each level and the roles and responsibilities of all the different people involved (e.g. Regional Treasurer, Area Administrator, District Pharmaceutical Officer, Area Chief Ambulance Officer). Both the structure itself and the language in which it is described are complicated. The organisation described above became operational on 1 April 1974. The main features of the organisation are shown in Figure 15.1.

When he first enters practice the relationship between Health Care Planning Teams, District Management Teams (DMT) and Sector

Figure 15.1: Organisation of the National Health Service since 1 April 1974

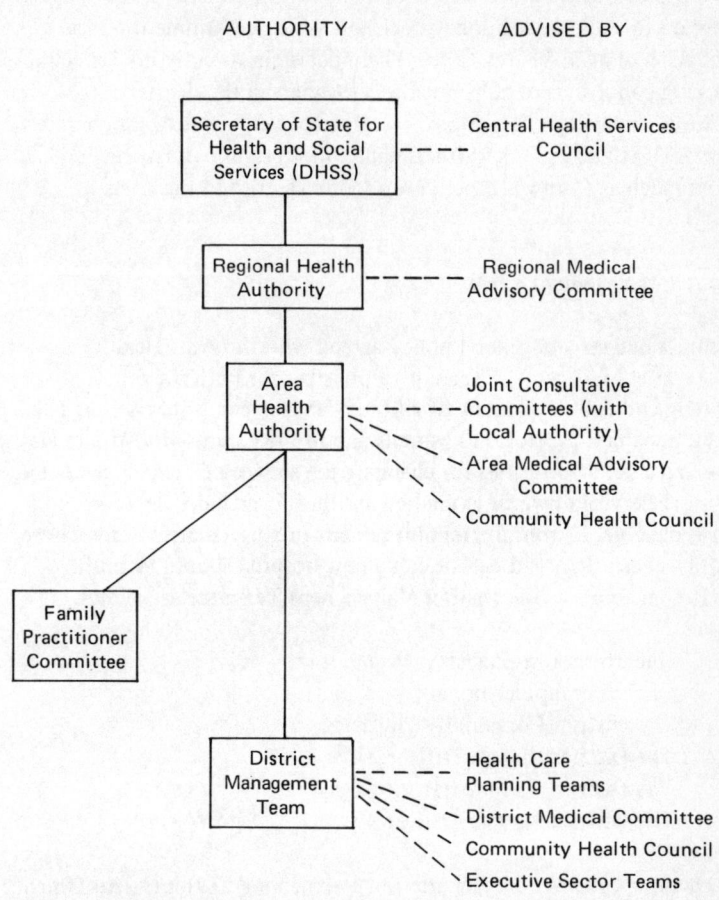

AUTHORITY   ADVISED BY

Secretary of State for Health and Social Services (DHSS) — — — Central Health Services Council

Regional Health Authority — — — Regional Medical Advisory Committee

Area Health Authority — — — — Joint Consultative Committees (with Local Authority)

Area Medical Advisory Committee

Community Health Council

Family Practitioner Committee

District Management Team — — — Health Care Planning Teams

District Medical Committee

Community Health Council

Executive Sector Teams

Management Teams (SMT) are unlikely to worry the young general practitioner with his mortgage, his new practice and young family, but the work of these committees directly affects all general practitioners. They do this by making policy decisions which determine the local allocation of available resources. These decisions directly influence the working conditions of all general practitioners in the district.

While most Regions contain several Areas, and most Areas contain several Districts, in some of the smaller, more rural parts of England and Wales (such as Cornwall) there is only one District to the Area.

District Management Team

Within a budget and general policy agreed with the Area Health Authority, the District Management Team is responsible for both the day-to-day running and future planning of all the NHS services in its district. This includes capital projects in hospitals and in the community. It includes agreeing a list of priorities for changing the service offered, such as running one service down or extending another. It includes decisions on a range of subjects from the reimbursement of a psychiatric nurse whose coat has been damaged to whether a new hospital should be built.

The members of the District Management Team are as follows:

(1) One hospital specialist.
(2) One general practitioner.
(3) The District Community Physician.
(4) The District Nursing Officer.
(5) The District Administrator.
(6) The District Finance Officer.

Of the six members there are four 'permanent' appointments (finance officer, administrator, nursing officer and community physician); of the three doctors on the District Management Team two are clinicians.

The general practitioner and the hospital specialist on the District Management Team are elected by the District Medical Committee from among their own members. This committee, the District Medical Committee, usually has between 12 and 16 members. It is composed of hospital specialists and general practitioners in equal numbers. In some districts, there is a representative of the dentists and other professional workers within the Health Service on this committee, as well as doctors representing a special interest or group. The general practitioner members of the District Medical Committee are themselves elected by their Local Medical Committee. As will be seen in the section on 'negotiations', Local Medical Committees have a medico-political function but it is also their responsibility to appoint representatives to the many committees involved in running the Health Service at AHA and district level.

The District Management Team takes advice, not only from its own members and their staff, but also from two other groups. The first group comprises *Health Care Planning Teams.* These are set up by the DMT to look into the requirements of special groups or at specific developments usually under the chairmanship of the District Community Physician. There may be a team for child care, another for services to the elderly. There may be a third to look into the running of the hospital transport system.

The second group of advisers are *Sector Executive Teams.* These are set up by District Management Teams when they consider they need co-ordinated advice concerning one particular part of the Health Service. There may, for example, be a Community Sector Team, a Mental Illness Sector Team, and a District General Hospital Sector Team. These are staffed by representatives of the professionals who work in the sector together with finance and administrative officers. The energy and enthusiasm with which Health Care Planning Teams and Sector Management Teams approach their work depends almost entirely on the individuals involved.

The Family Practitioner Committee

Although the previous section may seem to many to be of only theoretical interest, the one part of the Health Service organisation with which all general practitioners come in close contact throughout their professional careers is the Family Practitioner Committee. It is to this Committee that the general practitioner applies to be appointed as a principal in general practice. It is with this Committee that he signs his contract.

The Family Practitioner Committee is an agent of the AHA. Its powers are delegated to it by statute. It administers the Health Service arrangements, not only of general practitioners but also of the opticians, pharmacists and dentists who work within the Health Service in the community as independent contractors.

For the general practitioner the FPC is the direct point of contact with the administration of the Health Service. For many general practitioners who are not involved in committee work it may be their only point of contact. It is the FPC which appoints him as a principal. It is the FPC which pays him. It is through the FPC that a general practitioner receives the medical records of patients when they sign on with him; it is to the FPC that he returns these records when patients leave or die.

The Family Practitioner Committee is the direct successor to the body known before the 1974 reorganisation as the Executive Council. (This explains why the numbers of many forms in use in practice are prefixed by EC. More recent ones are prefixed by FP.) The FPC administrator is a member of the Area Health Authority staff. The appointment of the members of the FPC are made as follows:

By the	—Area Health Authority	11 members
	—Local Authority	4 members
	—Local Medical Committee	8 members (7 general medical practitioners, 1 ophthalmic medical practitioner)
	—Local Dental Committee	3 members
	—Local Pharmaceutical Committee	2 members
	—Local Optical Committee	2 members

So that, of the 30 members, 15 are appointed by the professions and 15 are laymen. The chairman is elected by the FPC from among its own members.

The areas and population served by different Family Practitioner Committees vary enormously, the smallest being Powys with a population of 100,000 — the largest being Kent with a population of 1,490,000.

Medical Practices Committee

The size of population and the number of practitioners in any one area are governed by many factors. In terms of cost of living, quality of life, the availability of good concerts, theatres and schools, each general practitioner will have his own priorities. But some parts of the country are more attractive to a larger number of general practitioners than other parts. In one area there may be an average of 1,600 patients to each general practitioner, in another there may be 3,000. In deciding to

appoint a doctor to a practice the FPC is governed by the recommendations of the Medical Practices Committee. This is a national committee
which, among its other functions, classifies each locality into one of
four different categories:

(1) *Designated areas:* which are under-doctored and to which
doctors are encouraged to go by various grants and payments (see
Chapter 8). Average list size in a designated area is over 2,500 patients
per doctor.

(2) *Open areas:* in which the number of doctors is below the recommended number. In these areas a general practitioner can usually
'put up his plate', but he attracts no special allowances. Average list size
in an open area is 2,200-2,500 patients per doctor.

(3) *Intermediate areas:* in which the total number of general
practitioners is considered adequate. Usually a general practitioner can
only enter practice in an intermediate area if another general practitioner
retires. Average list size in an intermediate area is 1,800-2,200 patients
per doctor.

(4) *Closed (restricted) areas:* in which the number of patients per
doctor is well below the national average. Close scrutiny is given to the
necessity of appointing a further general practitioner if one retires.
Average list size in a closed area is less than 1,800 patients per doctor.

The Medical Practices Committee meets in London on two days each
week. There are nine members appointed by the Secretary of State of
whom one is a lay member, one is a barrister, and seven are general
practitioners. In deciding whether an additional doctor may be appointed
or not in a particular district, the Medical Practices Committee does not
rely on rigid criteria of average list size alone. They may exercise their
discretion to take account of other factors such as the age of the doctors
in the district and in the practice, the number of temporary residents
seen or the number of outside appointments held. Many other considerations besides type of area and size of population influence their decision.

The Red Book

Although there are great differences between different types of practice
in different settings, the provisions of the Red Book apply to all.

Throughout this chapter and previous ones frequent reference has
been made to the Red Book, the correct name of which is *Statement of*

Fees and Allowances Payable to General Practitioners in England and Wales. General practitioners as a whole have taken a long time to realise that in spite of its tedious language and convoluted style understanding of the Red Book is essential to the efficient running of a practice.

For the administrative staff of the FPC, also, the Red Book is more than Chairman Mao's equivalent. It contains, not broad generalisations, but detailed criteria. It governs their daily actions. A copy is issued to each general practitioner by the FPC when he enters practice and is available free to all trainees. It lays down the conditions which have to be fulfilled before any fees or allowances can be claimed from the Family Practitioner Committee. The main sections of the Red Book can be summarised as follows:

(1) Paras. 1-10: general section: definitions of terms and list of current fees and allowances.

This section is updated when necessary, usually following recommendations made by the Review Body on Doctors' and Dentists' Remuneration.

(2) Paras. 11-60: payments to practitioners providing unrestricted medical services.

This section includes criteria which have to be met before payment is made and methods of applying for payment for all the different services. There are allocated paragraphs on everything from payments for out-of-hours responsibilities (paras. 22-24) and arrangements for prolonged study leave (para. 50), to reimbursement of part of the salaries of ancillary staff (para. 52). For the majority of general practitioners provisions within this section will govern the income which they will receive from the Health Service. A more detailed analysis will be found in Chapter 8.

(3) Paras. 61-70: payments to practitioners providing restricted services or with limited lists.

These paragraphs apply to the small number of general practitioners who have less than 1,000 patients registered with them or who only contract for certain defined services.

(4) Paras. 71-80: calculation of lists and arrangements for payment.

This section lays down the procedure followed by Family Practitioner Committees for payment and 'advance' payments to general practitioners. It also defines the procedure to be followed for appeals by general practitioners against decisions by the Family Practitioner Committee.

Negotiations between the Profession and the Government

Alteration of the Schedules of the NHS Regulations is by Act of
Parliament. Alterations in the Red Book are made by negotiation
between representatives of the profession and the DHSS. Amendments
to the Red Book when agreed are published as numbered pamphlets
labelled SFA (Statement of Fees and Allowances) and are distributed
to all appointed general practitioners and trainees in general practice
through Family Practitioner Committees. Amendments to the Red
Book are also made following recommendations of the Review Body —
if these are agreed by both Government and professions.

The Review Body itself was set up following the recommendations
of the Royal Commission on Doctors' and Dentists' Remuneration in
1960. The main aim was to avoid recurrent disputes about remuneration
by establishing an impartial body which would recommend just levels of
payment after hearing evidence from both Government and the profession. The Review Body is free to obtain additional information from
whatever source it wishes. It is free to decide its own methods of work,
the periods that its recommendations should cover, and how often to
undertake reviews. There are seven members and a chairman. In practice
in each of the past six years there has been one main review (published
in the Spring) supplemented by interim reviews when the need arose.

In addition to this formal review machinery, direct negotiations
between the profession and the Department of Health and Social
Security occur at regular monthly meetings. The general practitioners
who negotiate on behalf of the profession are appointed annually by
the *General Medical Services Committee* from among its members. The
GMSC currently (1980) has 80 members composed of elected and
appointed representatives. The majority of members (42) are general
practitioners who are elected by Local Medical Committees throughout
the country. A further six are elected annually by the conference of
Representatives of Local Medical Committees.

Local Medical Committees in turn are composed of general practitioners,
each of whom has been elected by fellow practitioners in his practice
district. So when it negotiates with the Government on terms and conditions of service the General Medical Services Committee represents
the interests of every general practitioner in the country, whether or
not he be a member of the BMA, RCGP, MPU or any other organisation.
Because the BMA is the only negotiating body for general practitioners
recognised by the Government, however, a typical British compromise
has resulted in the GMSC being recognised as a 'craft' committee within

the BMA (although some of its members may not be members of the Association).

The Royal Commission on the NHS

On 20 October 1975 the Government announced the appointment of a Royal Commission on the NHS with the following terms of reference: 'to consider in the interests both of the patients and of those who work in the National Health Service the best use and management of the financial and manpower resources of the National Health Service'. The Commission reported on the 18 July 1979. It put forward a number of proposals which would involve structural changes in the management of the Health Service in England (including the possibility of abolishing the level of Area management and setting up new District Health Authorities). The Government published its initial reactions as a consultative paper called *Patients First* in December 1979. It is due to issue firm proposals shortly (June 1980). Whatever form these proposals take it is unlikely that major changes will occur in the next two years — so the structure described in this chapter will probably survive for some time yet.

Summing Up

This chapter opened by pointing out the differences between practices, between practices in the same town, between practices in different locations. The rest of the chapter has shown that every practitioner in the Health Service, notwithstanding this diversity, works within the same broad framework. The same contracts, the same regulations, the same fees and allowances pertain to all.

Further Reading

Levitt, R. *Reorganised National Health Service*, 2nd edition (London: Croom Helm, 1977).
Management Arrangements for the Reorganised Health Service (London: HMSO, 1972).
Marks, J. *The Conference of Local Medical Committees and its Executive: An Historical Review* (London: General Medical Services Defence Trust, 1979).
Stevens, R. *Medical Practice in Modern England* (New Haven, Conn.: Yale University Press, 1966).

PART SEVEN: ORGANISATION

16 YOUR DAY, WEEK AND YEAR

It is no good having a highly organised practice if you yourself are completely disorganised. In fact the two are probably incompatible.

One often reads in the popular press about Dr Bloggs — a busy general practitioner, etc., etc. Busy often equals disorganised, as we can all appear as busy as we wish. This adjective 'busy' frequently appears to be a smoke screen produced by general practitioners to protect them from the demands of the public.

Over the past ten years or so one of the more obvious ways in which doctors have begun to organise themselves is reflected in the fall in home visiting and the decrease in surgeries held after 6 p.m. However, the management of time extends far beyond the manipulation of an appointment system.

Daily Routine

How the partners operate their surgeries depends on many factors, particularly the availability of consulting-rooms, patient demand, and other fixed commitments, such as clinical-assistant sessions.

Far too many doctors are fixed in the 9-10.30 a.m. and 5-7 p.m. surgery routine. If each partner has his own consulting-room then flexible timetables are possible. However, if consulting-rooms have to be shared then some thought will have to be given to the best way to organise this.

It is not a bad idea to have at least one partner consulting on the premises throughout most of the day. In this way a doctor is always on hand to deal with any crisis. This is a valuable back-up facility appreciated by his reception staff. Sessions during the course of the day can also be used for special clinics, such as antenatal, family planning, or geriatric screening clinics.

If one consulting-room is being used by two doctors, half-an-hour of 'dead time' between one surgery ending and the next beginning should always be allowed. Almost inevitably the first surgery will not be running exactly to time and there is no reason to stress the doctor further by the knowledge that he has to be out of the room promptly because it is needed by his partner.

Reception staff appreciate clear written instructions which state:

(a) The partners' daily and weekly timetable.

(b) The length of time of each surgery.

(c) The rate of booking required, e.g. eight patients per hour.

(d) The times when insurance medicals and similar items are to be booked, so that these can be arranged without constant referral back to the doctor.

(e) Instructions about receiving and accepting requests for visits. The procedure varies in different practices. It may be that the senior receptionist always deals with these requests or the doctor himself may wish to take the calls. The arrangement should be quite clear and the receptionist should know the details which she should obtain with each message.

(f) The on-call rota of doctors and ancillary staff.

On-call Rota

As the general practitioner's terms of service state that he is responsible for providing medical service for his patients seven days a week, it means that arrangements have to be made for someone always to be available for emergency calls.

A common arrangement is for all partners to take their own calls up until the end of morning surgery, and then for one partner to be available for emergency calls until the end of the evening surgery when the duty doctor for the night takes over.

Whatever rota is decided upon it is important that this is written down so that there is no argument as to who is responsible for taking a late call, and the receptionist should be informed of the whereabouts of the duty doctor throughout the day.

Meetings with Partners and Staff

It is wise to have a fixed time each day or week when the various members of the practice team meet. For instance, it is probably a good idea for the district nurse to see each partner daily to discuss new cases, as well as the changing requirements of patients under their shared care. In a health centre, or premises where she has her own room, this communication is, of course, much easier.

The health visitor and social worker should see each doctor at a fixed time at least once a week to catch up on the various cases. There do not have to be lengthy discussions but these meetings enable everyone to keep in touch with what is happening and certainly prevent any one member of the team from feeling isolated.

Ideally partners should meet each morning over coffee for discussion. However, varying commitments and timetables often mean that one doctor has finished his surgery and is anxious to get away, while another is still consulting, so these meetings do not always occur. In a small practice the partners normally see each other frequently enough to avoid any breakdown in communication, but some thought should be given to this in larger practices. As mentioned elsewhere a regular partnership meeting at least once a month should be arranged in addition to these more informal sessions.

It is particularly important that if one partner is about to take on an extra responsibility, be it a clinical-assistant session or chairmanship of the District Management Team, this matter is discussed fully and freely between the partners before any decision is taken. If the work takes place during practice hours then any income from the work should go into the partnership account and in this way friction is avoided. When the extra commitments are not producing any income, for example, serving on the LMC, then all partners should agree to the arrangement.

When all partners can either share an extra commitment, for example, teaching trainees, or each have a special interest of their own, it is an even better way of avoiding some members of the practice feeling that they are being 'put upon'.

Trainee Responsibility

If a trainee works in the practice then he too should have a written timetable which includes a statement of his teaching sessions with his trainer. Again the reception staff should know how he is to have his patients booked, and what arrangements have been made for his being on call and off duty. Appendix K contains the instructions which are given to trainees when they join one of the authors' practices.

The Week

When all these facts are taken into account, the whole of the working week should be clearly structured. The receptionists should have their own instructions as to when to book surgeries, who is on call at any time, and should have no doubt about the procedure they should follow.

Table 16.1: A Typical Weekly Timetable for a Three-partner Practice with only Two Consulting-rooms

	9-10.30 a.m.	11-1 p.m.	2-3.30 p.m.	4-6 p.m.	Evening/Night Duty
Mon	Dr A) Dr B) Surgery Dr C — Clinical-assistant session	Dr A) Dr B) Visits	Dr A — Ante-natal clinic Dr B — Insur-ance medicals	Dr B & Dr C — Surgery	
Tues	Dr B — Visits Dr A) Dr C) Surgery	Dr B — Surgery Dr A) Dr C) Visits	Dr A — Half-day Dr C — Ante-natal clinic, well woman clinic, FPA session	Dr B — Surgery	Dr C
Wed	Dr A) Dr B) Surgery Dr C — Visits	Dr A) Dr B) Visits Dr C — Surgery	Dr B — Half-day	Dr A & Dr C — Surgery	Dr A
Thurs	Dr A — Anaesthetic session Dr B) Dr C) Surgery	Dr B) Dr C) Visits	Dr B — Ante-natal clinic Dr C — Half-day	Dr A & Dr B — Surgery	Dr B
Fri	Dr A) Dr C) Surgery Dr B — Insur-ance medicals	Dr A) Meeting Dr B) with Dr C) Practice Team & visits	Dr B — Surgery	Dr A & Dr C — Surgery	
Sat	Drs A, B and C in rotation				

Monday: Dr A on call from 11 a.m. to 2 p.m. Dr C on call from 2 to 6 p.m.
Tuesday: Dr C on call from 11 a.m. to 3 p.m. Dr B on call from 3 to 6 p.m.
Wednesday: Dr A on call 11 a.m. to 6 p.m.
Thursday: Dr B on call 11 a.m. to 6 p.m.
Friday: Dr C on call 11 a.m. to 6 p.m.
Each doctor in rotation does 1 in 3 Monday and Friday evening and Saturday/Sunday duty.

The Year

The main planning for the year involves the arrangement for partners and staff holidays. In a theoretical three-partner practice not more than one partner should be on holiday at a time and probably some, if not all, of the partners will want time off during school holidays. If each partner is to have six weeks' holiday, which is fairly average now, then eighteen weeks of the year will see the practice working with two partners only. This means that a different, amended, timetable has to be produced for holiday periods or else a locum is employed to take the place of each partner in the timetable in turn.

Many drug firms now produce large wall charts showing a whole year at a time, and these are very useful for this type of planning. If different colours are used for each partner then these can be marked on the chart for the holiday periods to avoid overlap. Staff holidays can be incorporated on the same chart using different colour codes. It is important that the partners agree in advance who is to have first choice of dates for the year, and that all are agreed on the various holiday entitlements, study leave and sabbatical leave.

It is not intended that this chapter should imply that each doctor must have a rigid timetable to be strictly adhered to at all times irrespective of other considerations. Each doctor must consider his own priorities and incorporate them into his week accordingly. However, with an increasing number of doctors working with more partners and staff it is important that all concerned with the practice are aware of their responsibilities and are also aware of what other members of the practice are doing each day. Only in this way will confusion and arguments be avoided.

We are aware that much of the advice in this chapter is a repetition of advice given elsewhere. This is inevitable. The practice timetable whether over a short or long period reflects the way the practice is organised and the principles of management which form the subject of this book.

17 THE TRAINING PRACTICE

Over the past decade the number of practices involved in training has increased dramatically. The number of practices recognised for vocational training has doubled in the past five years, and with the advent of mandatory vocational training is unlikely to diminish. A period in general practice is now considered an essential part of the curriculum in most medical schools. Increasingly the training of community nurses, health visitors and social workers involves periods in the community attached to selected practices.

These developments have inevitably affected training practices in various ways. This chapter discusses the benefits and ill-effects which may ensue, and offers guidance on the special points of organisation which are needed within a training practice.

In an established practice, with settled staff and partners, methods and patterns of work have built up over a period of time. The people involved have got to know each other and, it is hoped, have developed a common purpose and identity. They are used to each other. Into this comfortable atmosphere the introduction of a stranger can be a disturbing event. There is potential disruption of routine, of working methods and of relationships. There may on the other hand be positive benefits to the practice with the introduction of new ideas or with a critical eye being turned on what has become too cosy, slack or rigid.

The extent of these effects will depend on the type of visitor, the personality of the individual, the length of time the visitor stays and the extent to which his activities penetrate the organisation. A social work student for a day, a medical student for a week, a health visitor trainee attached for three months, or a medical trainee for a year, will have different effects and repercussions.

Short-term Attachments

These attachments which last from a short visit of a few hours to one of several weeks are of two main types. In the first type the visitor wishes to explore a particular feature of the practice (record systems, computers, premises). Such visits usually involve one member of staff and are made for a specific purpose. It is essential that the purpose of the visit should be clearly defined and that one particular member of staff should be made responsible for looking after the visitor. If such visits become regular or repeated they can become a burden, interfering with practice routine and disrupting the work of the staff members involved. It is necessary to recognise the resentment this may cause and to come to an agreed practice policy involving both partners and staff.

The second type of short-term visitor is usually someone who has little experience or different experience and wishes to increase his/her knowledge of British general practice. A medical student for a fortnight, an American or French doctor for a week, a social work student for one day or week or for a month or two. With this type of visitor, who is likely to be an 'observer' rather than a 'participator', it is also necessary to define the purpose of the visit—both for the practice and the visitor. A timetable, preferably written if more than one person is involved, can be made out so that everyone can know where the visitor is and what they are supposed to be doing. The programme will depend on the visitor and the purpose of the visit. Questions to be answered will be:

(1) Who has overall responsibility for the visitor?
(2) What experience should the programme include?

Responsibility: for day-to-day activities responsibility for the visitor will usually be taken by the practice member of a similar profession, e.g. health visitor for health visitor, practice nurse for practice nurse, doctor for medical student, with the doctors having overall responsibility for what goes on within their practice.

Experience: this will include decisions as to whom the visitor should observe and why. Should they observe office routine, should they be present on home visits or in consultations, should they look at the books, attend staff or partnership meetings? In making these decisions there are some guiding rules which if followed minimise upset to staff and patients.

(1) That persons being observed by the visitor must have agreed to be observed.
(2) That the privacy of patients in the consultation should not be breached unless there are clear reasons for doing so. The visitor should be introduced and the reasons for the visit explained (albeit briefly) to the patients.
(3) That decisions concerning participation of the visitor in partnership

business should be explicitly agreed by all the partners.

(4) That the time and effort taken in entertaining the visitor should be understood by colleagues. Adjustments of practice workload should be made if this is appropriate.

Long-term Attachments

A long-term visitor, although an observer at the beginning of the attach-ment, is likely to become a participator – the longer the attachment, the greater the participation. Greater participation involves greater penetration of the group activities. It involves relationships with staff and partners which are not just temporary and superficial. It involves relationships with patients. If the visitor is a doctor in training, it involves acceptance by the partnership as a colleague, part of whose training may include knowledge of intimate partnership matters. It is as important that the questions which pertain to a short-term attachment concerning responsibility for the visitor, the purpose of the attachment, and the experience needed should be answered. It is also as important that the 'teachers', whether they be staff or partners, should be willing to teach, should be given time within their workload to teach and that the patients' need for privacy is respected. But the dimension added by time and participation raises further questions, namely:

(1) the effect of trainees on patients;
(2) the effect of trainees on staff;
(3) the effect of trainees on the partners;
(4) the effect of trainees on the practice.

On Patients

(1) The use of the consultation as an opportunity for teaching is one way in which the presence of a trainee directly affects patients. All methods of teaching disturb the normal one-to-one aspect of the consult-ation. Whether the trainee is an observer, or the trainee conducts the consultation and the trainer is an observer, to the patient this is an abnormal situation, usually unwelcome. The degree of patient displeasure will depend on the relationship between doctor and patient, the personality and problem of the patient and whether he or she has grown used to the situation in a teaching practice. The use of tape-recorders and video-cameras as a teaching aid is also an intrusion into the patients' privacy – but one which experience shows is rarely resented by patients if they

understand the reasons it is being done.

(2) The presence of a trainee affects the continuity of care patients receive. In practices where patients normally see whichever doctor is available, the presence of a trainee adds another possibility of diminishing continuity. Instead of one to two, patients may see any one of three doctors in a two-man partnership. In practices where patients normally see their 'own' doctors, the probability of seeing their own doctor, and thus of continuity, is lessened.

(3) The presence of a trainee affects the personal nature of the care patients receive. This is another aspect of loss of continuity. When a practitioner who regularly sees his own patients, and whose patients expect to see him, becomes a trainer the introduction of a trainee may result in the trainer's personal commitment being diminished in the eyes of the patients. They may feel rejected.

On Staff

(1) For staff, particularly staff who have been with the practice a long time, the introduction of a trainee may also be a disturbing event. They may feel that the trainee has no real commitment to 'their practice', that he is a bird of passage. With attachments for a few months, particularly in schemes where trainees are attached to several practices in succession in order to broaden their experience, the staff may scarcely have adjusted to the habits and personality of one trainee, when they are asked to accommodate another.

(2) With a trainee in the practice the workload of staff may increase considerably. In day-to-day practice there is little time for the trainer to explain all the minutiae of practice organisation to each trainee. The majority of questions as they arise will inevitably be dealt with by the staff—where are the forms, when does the blood go to the laboratory and how, when do we get X-ray results? These questions expand into practice policies—who tests the urines, when are swabs taken, how do I best arrange a course of desensitising injections, what is the practice policy for pill checks? Again, unless the trainee is to be eternally bombarding his trainer with such questions, the staff will answer most of them. They may well find themselves being asked to explain practice policies which they themselves do not understand.

(3) The task of arranging the appointment list for consultations with a trainee largely falls on receptionists. They are responsible for explaining to patients that they will be seeing the trainee rather than their own doctor and will at times have to use diplomacy when exposed to the patients' reactions after seeing 'the new doctor'.

On the Partners

(1) Although the initial impact of a trainee on the way the partners practise will be felt by his trainer, as he sees patients from the other partners their habits also will come under scrutiny. The teacher is aware from the beginning that inevitably his consultations, his methods, diagnostic ability and records will all be under scrutiny. It may only slowly dawn on the other partners that the trainee is forming an opinion of their abilities also. Such realisation can give rise to anxiety and possibly unhappiness between colleagues. The stranger may be looked on as a spy.

(2) This uncertainty may give rise to difficulties within the partnership as to how much the stranger should be allowed to see. There may be disagreements over the trainee's presence at partnership meetings where sensitive matters are discussed. There may be reluctance to open the books.

On the Practice

(1) The overall effect of a long attachment on a practice will inevitably largely depend on the personality and ability of the trainee, and whether this meshes satisfactorily or unsatisfactorily with the practice identity and ability. In addition there are two main considerations. On the one hand, the anxieties and extra work involved for staff and partners will tend to exaggerate and show up any tensions which exist, between partners, between staff, between partners and staff, between patients and practice. On the other hand, the presence of an enquiring stranger within the practice is a potent factor for inducing change. If records are poor, if practice management is faulty, if questions cannot be answered, if gaps are exposed, the stimulus to make changes increases.

(2) Organisation within the practice itself must include accommodation of the stranger. For trainees this increasingly means a separate consulting-room for their use. It means provision of an emergency case, equipment, books. It may also mean advice and help with living accommodation. It means space to park their car.

In summary, the presence of a stranger in the camp will inevitably have effects on a practice and on all those involved. The good effects can be enhanced and the disturbing effects minimised if both staff and partners are aware in advance of the considerations involved. It is equally important that the visitor is aware of the effects his/her presence will have.

CONCLUSION: CHOOSING A PRACTICE

Variety's the very spice of life,
That gives it all its flavour.

William Cowper

Choosing a practice has been likened to choosing a marriage partner and
indeed there are a number of similarities. If the choice is successful then
the relationship can be long, happy and rewarding, both emotionally and
financially. If the choice is incompatible then the results can be
disastrous with acrimony, unhappiness, and considerable financial loss
on all sides.

Therefore, a great deal of thought and care must go into choosing a
practice and partners who suit your particular temperament and family
needs. Most young doctors have a fantasy of the ideal practice. It would
be in a pleasant area, near the sea and good recreational facilities but
with a first-class district general hospital at hand and in premises bulging
with modern gadgetry and ancillary staff! Indeed a survey of vocational
trainees undertaken a few years ago showed that a large percentage
hoped for a medium-sized market-town practice with purpose-built
premises in a rural part of the country. Unfortunately, there are not
enough ideal practices around to suit everybody and this fantasy must
be tempered by reality.

There is a great deal to be said for young doctors gaining experience
of different types of practice before committing themselves. This
experience can be obtained either in a trainee year in general practice
(when the whole time does not have to be spent in one practice), or
by doing a variety of locums in different areas and types of practice.
If possible, it is worth trying to spend some time in groups, and also in
single-handed practice; there are considerable differences between the
two which are difficult to appreciate unless both have been experienced.

The single-handed practice is becoming less common. The present
trend, encouraged by government, is towards group practice. However,
there will always be a place for the individual practitioner in parts of
the country where the population is not dense enough to support
more than one doctor. There are also those doctors who, by temperament, are better suited to single-handed practice.

A group practice provides more variety of experience amongst the
doctors and decreases the risk of professional isolation. Duty rotas in

193

groups mean that a doctor is less frequently on call, but usually when on duty he is busier because of the larger number of patients for which he is responsible.

In a very large practice the incoming doctor may find it difficult to 'make his mark'. He may find himself having to bow to majority verdicts in practice decisions which may frustrate him if there are certain aspects of the practice which he would like to change.

In choosing a practice a difficulty which may seem surprising is the wide range of possibilities that the aspiring general practitioner has to choose from. But if during training the doctor has had experience of a variety of types of practice – urban, rural, single and groups – he should have some idea of the type and location of practice in which he is interested. A check list of the main factors which vary between one practice and another is given in Appendix L. Reference to this list may help to define priorities.

When the search for a practice begins, the best source of information is still the 'bush telegraph'. Chance enquiries started in this way can often bear fruit. This is particularly true for trainees on three-year vocational courses, because they have ample opportunity to meet local general practitioners during their stay in an area and their general practitioner trainer may also know of local vacancies. Course organisers, too, receive enquiries from local general practitioners seeking new partners.

Other services include advertising in the *British Medical Journal (BMJ)*, and in the *Journal of the Royal College of General Practitioners (JRCGP)* and in medical newspapers. The *BMJ* also runs a special service (The Medical Practices Bureau) for members to find practices and it is worth writing to Tavistock Square for the latest details of practices in specific localities. Not all the practice vacancies on their records are advertised in the *BMJ*. The local BMA offices are also always very helpful, and willing to give advice about vacancies.

One of the fascinations of visiting practices is that they are all so different. It is impossible to do anything more than generalise about the points to consider. However, the prospective partner might like to consider some of the following items:

1. The Partners. What are their ages and interests? How do they relate to each other and to you? Do they seem flexible in their ideas and not unwilling to modify their attitudes and habits if a good case can be made for doing so? Have there been any recent partnership changes and, if so, why? Indeed, why has the practice vacancy arisen at all?

Are the partners members of the Royal College of General Practitioners and, if not, what are their attitudes to the College? Are any of the partners trainers in a vocational training scheme? If not, are they at all interested in teaching? If there is a trainee in the practice, it would be certainly worthwhile trying to get him on his own to talk about the practice. Not many doctors are interested in research or in writing learned papers but if a partner is involved in research or has written papers then it again suggests that the practice may accommodate flexible interests. Do they have other outside interests, for example, medico-political, college activities, or Rotary?

In the past, the term 'senior partner' often meant not only the oldest member of the practice but also the doctor who had the right of veto in practice activities. He might have less out-of-hours work and take the greatest share of the profits. This is less so now, and the term 'senior partner' usually only refers to the doctor who has been in the practice the longest. It is important to see that a retirement clause is written into the partnership agreement so that the situation does not arise whereby an elderly doctor, out of touch with reality, refuses to retire. This clause should be written in such a way that, if the retiring partner wishes to go on working, he can then be re-employed, perhaps on a salary basis with less work and responsibility.

2. The Premises. Are they in a health centre or privately owned, purpose-built or adapted? If privately owned, what financial commitment will the incoming partner have to meet? If the premises seem inadequate, are there possibilities of addition, alteration or removal to more suitable ones in the future? Does each doctor have his own room and, if not, does the timetable of the practice allow each doctor to run his surgery within a reasonable period of time without too much pressure to vacate the room for the next doctor? Does the practice have a nurse and if so has she an adequate treatment-room? What is the practice policy about items of equipment, such as the ECG or basic furniture? Does the practice have a library? If so, are the books about general practice? Look at the records as they can reveal much about the practice's standard of medical care.

3. The Workload. Is the work shared evenly between the partners, including the rota duties? If partners have special commitments, such as clinical assistantships, who covers the practice while they are away? If one partner consults at a rate of, say, 12 per hour and another partner consults at a slower rate, will this cause argument and mis-

understanding? What holiday arrangements are made? It is usual now
for partners to have about six weeks holiday a year and this may or may
not include study leave. Some practices now also include arrangements
in their agreements for sabbatical leave, for example, six months every
eight years. This is a subject worth discussing. When a partner is on
holiday, are there adequate arrangements for covering his work?

4. Parity. The average length of time until parity of income is achieved
is usually about three years with an agreed percentage sliding scale until
this time. For example, in a three-man practice an incoming partner
might start at 25 per cent for the first year, 28 per cent for the second
year and 30 per cent for the third year with an equal one third share after
this. Some doctors resent the concept of working towards parity, but one
must remember that the other partners have built up the practice and
the incoming doctor reaps the benefit. Attitudes are perhaps easier to
understand if one remembers that twenty years ago it was not uncommon
for young partners to wait ten years or more for parity! As a general
rule it tends to be the case that popular practices in a pleasant area can
ask an incoming partner to work more time to parity than would be
expected in an overstretched city centre practice. It is normal for a new
entrant to a practice to work for a specified period of time, anything
from three months to a year, with an easy break clause in the contract.
This is to the advantage of both sides. It means that if it is mutually
agreed that the appointment was a mistake, then separation is easier.
This initial period may be in the form of a salaried assistantship or
partnership.

5. Partnership Agreements. All partnerships should have an agreement,
if only to be agreed and put away. The various aspects of this agreement
have been discussed in Chapter 11. Beware of the partnership which
says, 'Oh, we don't need an agreement!'

6. Income. Money has been dealt with in detail in Chapter 10. It has
been deliberately left low in the order of priorities when considering a
practice. If income is the only matter of interest then probably the young
doctor will be seeking a post overseas and not reading this book!
Naturally money is important, but too much emphasis can be laid upon
it. The average income of a well-trained new entrant to practice will
probably be in the region of £7,000 to £10,000 in the first year (1980
figures). It is essential to have a look at the practice accounts and get
some idea of the potential income of the practice and what earnings will

be at parity rather than be over-concerned with the starting figure. Enquire about the distribution of non-NHS earnings, such as private examinations, cremation fees, factory appointments, clinical assistant-ships, and so on. The fairest way is for all the practice income to be pooled and divided equally amongst the partners according to their shares. Any other method may lead to problems and even to the break-up of the partnership unless all partners feel happy with the arrangements. Nevertheless, it is quite common for partners to keep their own seniority award, and vocational training allowance. However, if this happens, it is important to see that no ill-will occurs as a result.

7. Housing. This will vary according to need but it is as well to have some idea of how much a suitable house in the area would cost. It is worth enquiring whether it would be possible to rent accommodation for some months while settling into the practice and getting to know the area. Some practices like the junior partner to live on the premises and although this habit is now dying out, it is as well to be aware of it.

8. Schools. Doctors with present or future young families forget that children need schools surprisingly quickly. Unless children are to be sent to boarding schools it is important to look at the local primary and secondary schools to find out what they have to offer.

All these points will need to be discussed when the doctor goes to the practice for an interview. However, before this stage he will need to write to the practice concerned either applying for the post or asking for further details. In doing this it is important to create a good impression. Handwriting should be legible and a typed curriculum vitae is preferable. The curriculum vitae should be fairly brief with a mention of secondary education and medical school. Give more detail about postgraduate experience indicating special qualifications where appropriate (e.g. FP certificate). State if married, wife's occupation (if any) and family (if any). Finally add hobbies and special interests (non-medical) since these help to build a more complete picture of you as an individual.

References will be required and these should be carefully selected. If a general practitioner knows you well, for example a trainer or family doctor, then use him. General practitioners tend not to be over-impressed with vague references from grandiose consultants in teaching hospitals. Remember to contact your referees to ask their permission to use their names. It is also useful to referees if you give them a quick outline of the practice to which you are applying.

Having been short-listed and asked for interview, the procedure may now vary a little. Many doctors like to entertain prospective partners and their wives for the day as this is often the best way to assess each other in surroundings which are fairly informal. It is unwise for a married doctor not to have taken his spouse to the practice before the final decision is made and they should ask if they can do this if not invited to do so. Indeed a practice where the wife was not invited would be suspect. Try to meet all the partners on this visit and remember that you are assessing them and their practice as much as they are assessing you.

Most practices expect to pay interview expenses. If they are not offered enquire about them as it will give a guide to practice attitudes on finance.

After the first visit, if both sides are interested in pursuing matters further, at least one more visit will be needed before a decision is taken. Do not rush into making a hasty decision because the area seems attractive or the premises are good. The main thing that really matters is the compatibility of the partners and yourself. If this is wrong then it will never work out. If it is right then with goodwill on all sides almost any other problem can be resolved. When in doubt about particular aspects, keep making enquiries and do not try to ignore them in the hope that they will go away. They never do.

Women General Practitioners

We are aware that this chapter has been written from the viewpoint of a young male doctor looking for a practice – and that a woman entering general practice would have other considerations and different priorities. Certainly the presence or absence of flexibility of practice arrangements, together with a willingness of the partners to contemplate changes, would rate highly on the check list of any married woman with a young family. Although the number of women entering full-time general practice is at present small, the position is likely to change. The number of women entering medical school is approaching that of men and the number of women starting vocational training for general practice is increasing steadily. We judge that this chapter will have to be rewritten should a further edition be contemplated.

APPENDIX A

Tabular presentation of comparison between the characteristics of independent contractors and salaried employees in bureaucracies

Characteristic	Independent Contractor	Salaried Employee
1. General characteristic	Variety Self-employed Administratively untidy Variable standard of service	Uniformity Employee Administratively tidy 'Master/servant' order
2. Sociological classification	Burgess	Some are spiralists
3. Authority	General—often employs staff Can never be given orders Negotiators	Specific—accountable upwards and authority over subordinates 'Officers/supervisors'
4. Philosophy	Flexible and great freedom to negotiate local arrangements	Rules, often nationally determined Consistency and standard-isation of policy
5. Personality of operator	Individuality encouraged Use of names and relation-ships with clients valued	Individuality discouraged Anonymity of staff Correspondence to junior members of hierarchy discouraged
6. Contract	Contract for services	Contract of service
7. Pay	Usually not incremental salary scale Often some element of fee for service or commission	Salary by definition Usually incremental scale
8. Premises and equipment	Usually responsible for providing own premises	Usually provided by the employing authority
9. Staffing	Usually responsible for own holidays, locum, and pension	Employer responsible for holiday arrangements, locums, and often pension
10. Retirement	Variable Individual negotiation	Usually compulsory at fixed age

11. Partnership(s)	Common 'Jointly and severally' responsible in law and for tax and partners' debts	Rare No responsibility for colleagues' taxes or debts
12. Income tax assessed under	Schedule D 'wholly and exclusively'	Schedule E, PAYE 'wholly and necessarily'
13. Responsibility	Ultimately answerable to client/patient	Ultimately answerable to superior or employer
14. Professional negligence	Professional is solely responsible and alone can be sued	Employing authority responsible and can be sued (as well as or instead of professional)
15. Degree of choice by client/patient	Usually wide choice and relatively easy to change	Little or no choice of individual or department Difficult to change

Source: Gray, D.J. Pereira. 'General Practitioners and the Independent Contractor Status', *Journal of the Royal College of General Practitioners, 27* (1977), pp. 750-6.

APPENDIX B: EXAMPLES OF TEAMWORK

1. Child Care Surveillance

A plan for parents showing recommended times for appointments for child care surveillance – three-partner practice in Exeter

---

We like all the children in our practice to have a regular series of check-ups and immunisations.

The programme we are following is shown below and is the same or very similar to the programme at the clinics. Please bring your child's record of immunisation if you can.

Please always bring your child when you have each appointment. If for any reason you cannot come please *ALWAYS* let us know so that another child can be given the appointment.

Denis Pereira Gray Helen Chapman, Health Visitor
Ann Buxton
Russell Steele   D. Smith, Practice Sister

1. Birth or soon after Medical examination by doctor

2. Six weeks (usually at the same time as mother's postnatal examination) Medical examination by doctor

3. Six months Examination by health visitor. Immunisation by sister (Triple 1 and polio 1)

4. Eight months Hearing test by health visitor. Immunisation by sister (Triple 2 and polio 2)

5. 1 year birthday check Medical examination by doctor and health visitor
Measles injection by sister

6. Fourteen months Immunisation by sister (Triple 3 and polio 3)

7. 2 years Examination by health visitor

8. 3½ years Medical examination by doctor and examination by health visitor

9. 4½ years Pre-school immunisation (tetanus/diptheria) by sister

10. 9½ years Booster immunisation (diptheria/tetanus) by sister

11. 10½ years (girls only) Immunisation against german measles by sister

The check/immunisation due this time is number 1 2 3 4 5 6 7 8 9 10 11

Your appointment is at . . . . on . . . .

---

2. Care of Schizophrenic Patients in the Community

A written plan of care for practice sisters working in a general-practice treatment-room – three-partner practice in Exeter

---

Introduction. Schizophrenia now occurs in about one in a hundred of the population and is often controllable by chemical drugs of the phenothiazine group particularly fluphenazine (Modecate) or flupenthixol (Depixol) which is a slow-release preparation.

Aim. The aim is to maintain the patient at home and out of hospital.

Doses. If starting fluphenazine (Modecate) for the first time the test dose of 0.5ml (25mg per ml) should be given. The effects normally last between 15 and 40 days. Seeing all patients every three weeks is a reasonable regular routine but the patient's own doctor is responsible for deciding the exact frequency.

Prescriptions will be written as:

    a) Inj. fluphenazine (Modecate) 25mg every three weeks.
                      Mitte 10

    b) Inj. flupenthixol (Depixol) 20mg every three weeks.
                      Mitte 10

Precautions. Precautions should be taken about side-effects if key organs like the liver, heart or kidneys are failing. Not to be used in pregnancy.

Side-effects. Side-effects are the anti-cholinergic group and include drowsiness, lethargy, blurred vision, dry mouth, constipation, mild hypotension and Parkinsonian symptoms such as twitching or stiffness of muscles.

Care in the Treatment-room. 1. Ensure that each patient on fluphenazine has a card which never leaves the sister's box. Schizophrenic relapse occurs quickly once treatment is stopped so failure to attend means a follow-up appointment should be sent immediately and attendance is then checked by the sister.

    2. Give patients time in the consultation to talk about themselves and look particularly for the classic features of schizophrenia which are:
    (a) Muddled thinking.
    (b) Funny moods, i.e. too happy or too sad in relation to their situation or
         just not reacting emotionally.
    (c) Unreasonable suspiciousness (paranoia).
    (d) Look for side-effects of the drugs especially:
        (i) Odd movements of the tongue.
        (ii) Stiffness or twitching muscles especially the face.
        (iii) Odd movements in general.

    3. Ensure patient is seen by their own doctor at least every six months and at the same consultation if any of the above symptoms are present or if the sister just feels something is wrong.

4. Test urine once a year and record.

5. Take blood once a year—usually in the month of their birthday for:
   (a) Liver function
   (b) Blood urea

Procyclidine 5mg (Kemadrin). Procyclidine is used as an anti-Parkinsonian agent and is therefore often used with drugs like fluphenazine (Modecate) to counteract the tendency that these drugs have to produce Parkinsonism.

All doctors in the practice are now trying to reduce the prescriptions for this in order to avoid side-effects from the main drug being masked and will discuss this with any patient who queries the treatment.

3. Practice Policy: Oral Iron in Pregnancy

A prescribing policy for routine prescriptions and for iron and folic acid during pregnancy – three-partner practice in Exeter

British National Formula (1976-8) recommends daily supplement equivalent to 100mg elemental iron *plus* 300mcg folic acid.

NAME	IRON SALT	EQUIVALENT ELEMENTAL IRON VALUE	FOLIC ACID	Cap. or Tab.	Cost/100 MIMS May 77	
1. 'FECAP FOLIC'	Fe Sulphate 450mg	80mg	350mcg	cap.	£2.00	Too little
2. 'FE FOL Spansule'	Fe Sulphate 150mg	47mg	500mcg	cap.	£2.00	for a one daily
3. 'FER Folic'	Fe-gluconate 250 mg	30mg	500mcg	s-c tab.	0.94	dosage
						+ vitamins
4. 'FERROCAP-F'	Fe Fumarate	110mg	350mcg	cap.	£1.72	
5. 'FERROGRAD folic'	Fe sulphate 325mg	105mg	350mcg	tab.	£2.00	High cost
6. 'FOLEX 350'	Fe Fumarate 308mg	100mg	350mcg	s-c tab.	0.70	
7. 'IROFOL C'	Fe sulphate 325mg	105mg	350mcg	tc tab.	2.39	High cost
						+ ascorbic acid
8. 'PREGADAY'	Fe Fumarate	100mg	350mcg	fc tab.	1.00	
9. 'PREGFOL'	Fe Sulphate 270mg	86mg	500mcg	cap.	0.90	Too little
10. 'PREGNAVITE Forte F'	Fe Sulphate 252mg	76mg	360mcg	s-c tab.	0.60	iron for once
11. 'Slow FEFOL'	Fe Sulphate 160mg	52mg	400mcg	fc tab.	1.59	daily dosage

Assuming (previous practice policy decisions) that *once* daily dosage of *single tablet or capsule* is required then: 1, 2, 3, 9, 10 and 11 are ruled out as having too little iron. This leaves FOLEX 350 as the cheapest, in sugar-coated tablet form, PREG-ADAY as a film-coated tablet and FERROCAP-F as a capsule in order of cost as the preparations of choice. FERROGRAD folic and IROFOL C are excluded on basis of cost.

Recommendation. Practice policy to use PREGADAY as the preparation of first choice.

Buxton, A.
Personal Communication

APPENDIX C: PRACTICE NURSE ACTIVITIES

Annual workload of three part-time practice sisters working in the treatment-room of a three-partner practice in Exeter with 6,500 NHS patients

Diagnostic			1976	1977	1978	1979
	Measuring	blood pressure	372	308	305	357
		height	25	29	80	52
		weight	318	442	404	514
		peak flow	16	19	5	0
	Taking	blood	1,876	1,817	2,066	2,227
		high vaginal swabs	28	47	74	49
		skin scrapings	—	—	2	5
		throat swabs	13	8	18	42
		wound swabs	42	56	41	64
		ECG	—	—	—	24
		glucose tolerance	12	12	—	—
		tine test	20	17	23	36
		Total	2,722	2,755	3,018	3,370
Treatment		Bandaging (support)	74	96	53	97
		Cervical collar	—	—	—	13
		Dressings	1,082	916	876	1,003
		Ear syringe	261	257	251	363
		Foot care	149	169	163	227
		Injections—antibiotic	59	—	1	30
		Modecate & Depixol	242	364	280	254
		Myocrisin	—	—	—	58
		Other therapeutic	165	106	175	197
		Minor operations	18	39	31	29
		Pessary change	7	10	11	18
		Suture removal	162	157	165	199
		Wart painting	18	53	49	62
		Total	2,237	2,167	2,055	2,550
Assessment		Antenatal	24	22	149	200
		Check vaccination	36	15	29	18
		Diabetic care	37	72	46	48
		Ear checks	120	100	112	133
		Pill check	12	—	31	36
		Total	229	209	367	435
Preventive		Immunisation:				
		influenza	342	460	388	366
		paediatric	420	338	321	427
		prophylactic (cholera, tetanus)	325	491	415	712
		rubella	36	72	36	48

Preventive	1976	1977	1978	1979
hay fever prophylaxis	100	98	–	–
Help with IUD	34	26	65	55
	1,257	1,485	1,225	1,608
Miscellaneous	25	92	111	94
Total for year	6,470	6,708	6,776	8,057

APPENDIX D: SPECIMEN JOB INTERVIEW SHEET

	Comments
Date	
Application for post of	
Name . . . . Age	
Address	
Married/single . . . .?	Husband likely to be promoted or moved
Children . . . . .Ages	? Dependent. What happens when they are ill?
Present position	
Previous experience . . . .?	Relevant? how skilled
	? How much responsibility
Education	? Sheltered/exposed
Qualifications	
Jobs	? Frequent/ no changes
Reasons for leaving	
Reasons for applying	? Job satisfaction
	? Money ? Convenience
Health record	? Recurrent illness
General appearance/manner	
Salary	? Salary expected
Questions asked	? Overkeen on 'rights'
	? Slap-happy
Availability	? When free to start
References	? Relevant

At the end of the interview the following questions should be able to be answered:

How will he/she fit into the practice?
How will he/she get on with the existing staff?
How will he/she cope with the most unattractive part of the job?
Do I like the person?
Do I respect the person?

Grading: A. B. C. D.

APPENDIX E: AVERAGE PRACTICE INCOME 1975/6

Analysis of income of average GP principal 1975/6: calculated by taking total sum dispensed by Family Practitioner Committees and dividing by the number of general practitioner principals

1	Basic practice allowance	2,531.20
2	Supplementary practice allowance	484.12
3	Capitation fees: patients aged under 65 years	4,509.41
	" " " " patients aged 65-74 years	629.68
	" " " " patients aged 74 years and over	427.80
4	Supplementary capitation fees	586.43
5	Temporary residents up to 15 days	104.54
	" " " " " over 15 days	97.69
6	Contraceptive services	210.00
7	Vaccination and immunisation	161.44
8	Cervical cytology	24.74
9	Night visit fee	126.08
10	Maternity medical services	596.44
11	Arrest of dental haemorrhage	0.25
12	Emergency treatment fee	10.58
13	Anaesthetic fees	1.34
14	Vocational training allowance	21.59
15	Seniority allowance	634.23
16	Postgraduate training allowance	10.96
17	GP trainer allowance	236.08
18	Rural practice payments	210.71
19	Dispensing fees	974.38
20	Designated area allowance Type I	165.52
	" " " " " " " Type II	16.97
21	Initial practice allowance	15.50
22	Inducement allowance	11.76
23	Group practice allowance	294.88
24	Employment of assistant	9.45
25	Reimbursement—practice accommodation	570.43
	" " " " —ancillary staff	896.81
26	Women doctors retainer scheme	0.21
27	Additional payments during sickness or confinement	21.42
28	Prolonged study leave	2.31

Source: *Mims Magazine*, No. 35 (Nov. 1976), p. 92.   14,593.20

APPENDIX F: DISPENSING

Dispensing doctors represent approximately 10 per cent of general practitioners. Historically, most general practitioners provided their patients with advice and medicine. Under the National Health Service the system was continued whereby doctors who had registered patients living more than one mile from the central surgery were able to continue a dispensing service for these patients. For doctors in rural areas, where there was no chemist shop within one mile of the surgery, then all the patients could be on the dispensing list.

It has been argued by the pharmacists that dispensing doctors should have special training. It has also been argued that the existence of dispensing doctors threatens the survival of retail pharmacists in small communities. The Clothier Committee, which was set up in 1975 to 'find a solution which would secure sensible arrangements for the supply of prescription medicines in rural areas', reported in November 1977. Its main proposal was the establishment of a national statutory body to regulate what was called 'significant changes in dispensing arrangements in rural areas'. Meanwhile, a voluntary standstill has been agreed so that neither doctors nor pharmacists open fresh dispensing outlets without joint agreement. The general practitioner who dispenses may do so either under the capitation system or under a drug tariff system.

(a) The Capitation System

The capitation system requires the general practitioner to supply drugs required by his patients. For the cheaper common medicines he provides these from his stock. He is remunerated for this by the payment of an additional capitation fee in respect of each patient on his dispensing list. The current capitation fee for dispensing to patients (1980) amounts to 0.52p per annum. There are, in addition, a large number of drugs which are termed 'expensive' and are on a special list. The general practitioner may provide these himself, writing a special prescription form which is priced separately by the Prescription Pricing Authority and for which he therefore receives an additional payment from the Family Practitioner Committee. If the general practitioner does not have these particular medicines in his dispensary, the patient is given a green prescription

209

form FP.10(D), which he may take to any retail pharmacist.

(b) Drug Tariff System

Relatively few doctors dispense on the capitation system; most now use the drug tariff system. This system of payment basically requires the general practitioner to act in the same manner as a retail pharmacist towards his dispensing patients. He issues a white prescription form in the normal way for any medicine required by the patient. This prescription is then dispensed in the general practitioner's dispensary and at the end of each month the total number of forms collected by the doctor's dispensary are sent to the Prescription Pricing Authority for payment.

Retail pharmacists and doctors dispensing under the Drug Tariff system are paid for their services in broadly the same way. The differences are in respect of superannuation, broken pack allowance and additional payments for urgent prescriptions. In the case of the retail pharmacist a slightly higher on-cost percentage is allowed, but there are no superannuation benefits as there are for general practitioners. Pharmacists are allowed to claim additional payment where they may have to dispense a small quantity of a drug from a standard pack, and find themselves left with unwanted stock. For prescriptions which are required urgently by patients, especially those required out of hours, pharmacists can claim additional fees; these are not allowed in the case of dispensing family doctors.

The dispensing doctor has certain legal obligations. It is his responsibility to see that medicines are dispensed accurately and safely and that all the regulations of the various Drug Acts are conformed with. He may employ a qualified pharmacist who will be entitled to dispense medicines on his own responsibility, but more commonly the dispensing doctor employs a dispensing aide who works under the supervision of the general practitioner. In such circumstances, it goes without saying that the general practitioner is ultimately responsible for medicines dispensed and, in particular, for handling and checking all scheduled and dangerous drugs.

In a rural area, the general practitioner frequently has a relatively small list. The dispensing part of the practice may bring in an important proportion of the practice's income. As a rough guide, the 'profit' on dispensing should range from 12 to 20 per cent of the gross turnover. In part, it would depend on the additional staff costs and the care with which stocks of expensive medicines are controlled. In the special case of the doctor who is reimbursed under the capitation system, his profit from dispensing will depend largely on his prescribing habits. If he constantly 'over-prescribes' his net profit will be smaller.

Patients who are used to the system of receiving a prescription from their doctor and then taking it to a retail chemist for dispensing are often surprised and impressed by the service which patients registered with dispensing practices obtain. Not for them the need to wait to see the doctor and then wait at the chemist's to have their prescription made up, the two operations can be done in the same building usually at the same time. Dispensing doctors, too, have tremendous advantages over their non-dispensing colleagues; during out of hours duty they are able to provide patients with the full course of medicines required and do not have to provide supplies of emergency drugs for which they are not paid. Again, in rural areas, patients are grateful to the doctor who not only visits but at the same time leaves the necessary medicines in the patient's house. Such a service depends on particular circumstances, but often it is extremely satisfying to both doctor and patient.

(c) Personal Dispensing

For general practitioners who do not normally dispense it is possible to make a claim from the FPC on the drug tariff basis for certain vaccines, anaesthetics, injections and diagnostic reagents which he personally administers to patients. The practitioner buys the drug or reagent, administers it and claims on form FP34 (Doctors). Particulars of the drugs and payments allowed can be found under para. 44.13 and para. 44 schedules 1-4 in the Red Book.

APPENDIX G: MODEL EXPENSE FORM

Model form of income and expenditure account for use by general practitioners

Doctors . . . .

Income and Expenditure Account for the year ended . . . . 19 . . . . . .

Expenditure		Income	
Medical expenses		*Family Practitioner Committees*	
Drugs, dressing etc.	xx	Fees and other payments for	
Sundry Equipment etc.	xx	medical services including	
	xxx	dispensing	xxx
Premises		Reimbursements for:	
Rent (including paid to health		Premises (rented and owned	
centres)	xx	including health centres)	xx
Rates	xx	Ancillary help	xx
Fuel, light, power and water	xx	Trainees	xx
Telephones	xx	Locums	xx
Insurance (building and contents)	xx		xxx
Exterior and interior main-		*Local authorities and other*	
tenance and decorations	xx	*government departments*	
Cleaning etc.	xx	*etc.*	xxx
Interest (building society and		*Other (including private)*	xxx
other loans in connection			xxx
with purchase of premises		*Income assessed under*	
including interest on group		*Schedule E*	
practice loans)	xx	Net fees	xx
	xxx	PAYE deductions	xx
Staff costs (wages, national		Superannuation and other	
insurance and super-		deductions	xx
annuation contributions)			xxx
Assistants	xx		
Trainees	xx		
Dispensers, receptionists			
and other staff (including			
salaries relating to wives)	xx		
Staff advertising and agency fees	xx		
	xxx		
Locum and other deputising			
costs	xxx		
Car and travel			
Car rental	xx		
Tax and insurance	xx		
Petrol, oil and repairs	xx		
Taxi and other travel expenses	xx		
	xxx		

Other expenses

Postage	xx
Stationery, magazines and technical literature .	xx
Professional and other subscriptions	xx
Refresher courses and professional training	xx
Medical committee expenses	xx
Laundry and dry cleaning	xx
Accountancy and legal	xx
Bank interest and charges (not related to properties)	xx
Hire purchase charges	xx
Sundry	xx
	xxx

Depreciation and amortisation

Premises	xx
Cars	xx
Equipment	xx
	xxx
	xxx
Net income for the year	xxx
	£xxxx

£xxxx

Notes

1. It is important to ensure that payments received from FPCs in respect of part or complete reimbursement of expenses are shown as income and any deductions therefrom by way of health centre expenses, medical committee expenses, etc., shown as expenditure.
2. All expenses should include VAT attributable to that expense.
3. If more than one surgery is used it may be informative to show separately the premises expenses relating to each surgery.
4. It may be considered appropriate to make adjustments for private use of motor cars and house expenses in the accounts themselves rather than in the tax computations in which event it would probably be desirable to indicate this fact against the items concerned.

Source

Sub Appendix B to Appendix II, Report of the General Medical Services Committee to the Annual Conference of Representatives of Local Medical Committees.

APPENDIX H: PRACTICE FINANCIAL ANALYSIS FORM

Sample of analysis form used in a three-partner practice

INCOME

1977   1978

Head Counts
    Capitation fees.....................
    Temporary residents.................
    Contraceptive fees..................
        Total Head Counts.................... XX

Practice Allowances basic/supplementary........ XX

Item of Service
    Maternity fees......................
    Vaccination/immunisation............
    Cervical cytology...................
    Night visit fees....................
    Emergency treatment fees............
        Total Item of Service................. XX

Personal
    Seniority allowances................
    Vocational training allowance.........
    GP trainer allowance................
        Total Personal...................... XX

Type and Position
    Rural practice......................
    Group practice......................
    Dispensing..........................
        Total Type and Position................ XX

Sundries
    Total FPC payments...................... XX

Reimbursements
    Rent...............................
    Rates..............................
    Wages..............................
    Pension premiums...................
    NI.................................
    Trainees' salary/allowance.............
    Drugs and appliances................
        Total Reimbursements................. XX

Non-NHS Practice
    Insurance medicals..................
    Nat. Children's Homes...............

Private patients . . . .
Balance of analysis book . . . .
Dental anaesthetics . . . .
University . . . .
Others . . . .
    Total Non-NHS Practice   XX

TOTAL INCOME   XX

RUNNING EXPENSES

1977   1978

1. *Staff Costs*
   a. Wages: receptionist/secretary . . . .
                        nursing . . . .
                        cleaning . . . .
         Out of hours: partners' wives . . . .
                        others   XX
       Total   XX
            Medical: locum . . . .
                      trainee . . . .
       Total   XX
   b. National Insurance (Employers) . . . .
   c. Pensions: ancillary staff . . . .
                  partners' wives . . . .
       Total   XX
         Total Staff Costs   XX

2. *Cost of Premises*
   a. Rents: premises . . . .
                 for trainee . . . .
       Total   XX
   b. Rates: general . . . .
                 water . . . .
       Total   XX
   c. Repairs/redecorations . . . .
   d. Insurance (of premises) . . . .
       Total Cost of Premises   XX

3. *Servicing Costs*
   a. Telephones . . . .
   b. Heat and light . . . .
   c. Postage . . . .
   d. Printing and stationery . . . .
       Total Servicing Costs   XX

4. *Professional Costs*
   a. Accountancy . . . .
   b. Bank charges . . . .
   c. Subscriptions . . . .
   d. Journals, books . . . .
   e. Medical drugs/dressings . . . .
         Replacement equipment . . . .
   f. Partners'/trainees' superannuation . . . .

g. LMC levys . . . .
    Total Professional Costs   XX

5. *Sundries*
  General . . . .
  Miscellaneous . . . .
  Domestic . . . .
    Total Sundries   XX

TOTAL RUNNING COSTS   XX

CAPITAL EXPENSES

  Furnishing . . . .
  Office equipment . . . .
  Medical equipment . . . .
    Total Capital Costs   XX
                                      XX

TOTAL EXPENDITURE   XX

SUMMARY

1977   1978

  FPC income . . . .
  Reimbursements . . . .
  Non-NHS income . . . .
  Total Income

  Total expenses . . . .
  Available to partners . . . .
  Income tax paid . . . .
  Drawings by partners . . . .

  Practice Expense Analysis
  Gross expense per patient . . . .
  Reimbursements . . . .
  Net expense per patient . . . .

  Gross income per patient . . . .
  Net expense . . . .
  Net income per patient . . . .

APPENDIX I: THE NHS IN SCOTLAND

Although in the main the fees, allowances, terms and conditions of service are the same for general practitioners throughout Great Britain, the health services in Scotland have always operated under separate NHS Acts. In 1978 the various NHS Acts since 1947, including the NHS (Scotland) Act 1972 which corresponds to the Act which reorganised the NHS in England and Wales in 1974, were consolidated under the National Health Service (Scotland) Act 1978.

In the 1974 reorganisation 15 Health Boards were established in Scotland. These Boards are directly responsible to the Scottish Home and Health Department. Their responsibilities are broadly those which are carried out by Regional and Area Health Authorities in England and Wales. The Common Services Agency, which directly administers the Blood Transfusion Service and the Ambulance Service, provides services under the Scottish Home and Health Department for all Health Boards.

In ten Health Boards there are further subdivisions into two or more Districts because of size of population and/or geographical location. In the remaining five Health Boards there are no subdivisions. Each Health Board delegates administration concerning primary care to a General Medical Practitioner Committee which is composed of equal numbers of lay and medical members together with a lay chairman.

In contrast to the position in England and Wales where general practitioners have contracts with Family Practitioner Committees, each general practitioner in Scotland contracts his or her services to one or more Health Boards.

The medical advisory structure in Scotland is complex. The relationship between the main administrative levels and their advisory committees is shown in Figure AI.1. It will be noted that each Health Board is advised by its Area Medical Committee, a University Liaison Committee and by Local Health Councils. The Area Medical Committee consists of representatives of all Divisions within the Area. Each Area Medical Committee has a subcommittee for general practitioners (which usually has the same membership as the LMC) and most have subcommittees for other specialties.

In addition to advising its Health Board each Area Medical Committee is represented on the National Medical Consultative Committee. This Committee, which includes members from Royal Colleges and

Universities, has eleven specialty subcommittees. It is the function of the National Medical Consultative Committee (together with the National Consultative Committees of other professions working in the Health Service) to advise the Scottish Health Services Planning Council on matters of policy in relation to clinical provision. The Planning Council in turn advises the Scottish Home and Health Department.

One major difference between the organisation of the service in Scotland and the service in England and Wales is that in Scotland no clinician takes a direct part in local management decisions unless he is appointed to a Health Board by the Secretary of State. In England and Wales a general practitioner and hospital specialist are elected by their colleagues to be members of the District Management Team. In this way, clinicians in England and Wales are directly involved in planning and management decisions.

Another difference is that in Scotland there is no statutory recognition of any medical advisory committee below the level of the Area Medical Advisory Committee. The district medical committees that exist have no standing under the Act, unlike the District Medical Committees in England and Wales which have a defined composition and function.

It is to be noted that the consultative document *Structure and Management of the NHS in Scotland* (HMSO, 1979) proposes considerable changes in the administrative arrangements outlined above and invites suggestions for changes in the medical advisory structure. As in England and Wales, these matters are currently (1980) under discussion.

Figure AI.1

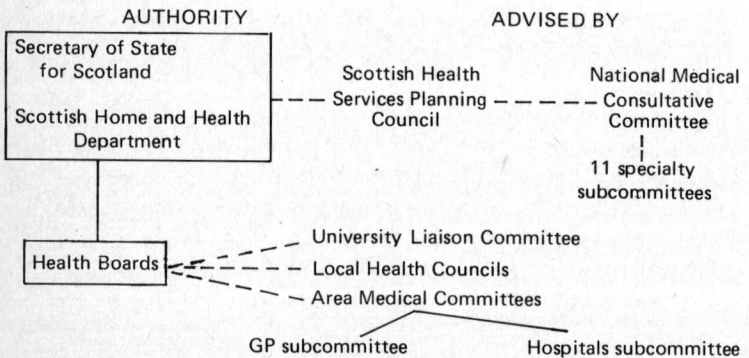

APPENDIX J: THE NHS IN NORTHERN IRELAND

In Northern Ireland the administration of the Health Service differs
from that found in both Scotland and in England and Wales. The main
difference is that in Northern Ireland there is integration between the
Health Service and Social Services Departments at all levels. Northern
Ireland is administered under a separate Act – the Health and Social
Services (Northern Ireland) Order 1972. The Health and Social Services
have a common budget and common planning procedures.

There are four Boards, called Health and Social Services Boards.
As in Scotland, there are no Family Practitioner Committees, and the
general practitioner is in contract with a Board (Health and Social
Services Board), although (as in Scotland) responsibility for the day-to-
day running of family practitioner services is in the hands of a Central
Services Agency acting on behalf of all four Health Boards.

In Northern Ireland, unlike Scotland, there are planning committees
at a district level which have statutory recognition. The District
Executive Committee in Northern Ireland is the equivalent of the
District Management Team found in England and Wales. The composition of the District Executive Committee is as follows:

(1) One doctor (clinician).
(2) One administrator (District Administrator).
(3) One nurse (District Nursing Officer).
(4) One community physician (District Community Physician).
(5) One social services worker (District Social Services Officer).

The 'clinical doctor' may be either a general practitioner or a specialist.
He is elected by the District Advisory Medical Committee. This differs
from the organisation in England and Wales where there are *two*
clinicians on the DMT – one a specialist, the other a general practitioner.
The inclusion of a social services worker is peculiar to Northern Ireland
and a reflection of the integration between the Health and Social
Services departments.

APPENDIX K: TRAINEE TIMETABLE

The whole essence of any timetable is that it should structure the time available to incorporate all the required activities. It should also be flexible to allow for the changing needs of the persons involved.

The following is a proposed, but negotiable, timetable and it will certainly change from time to time.

	9-11 a.m.	11-1 p.m.	2-4 p.m.	4-6 p.m.
Monday	Surgery	Discussion and visits	Project time and miscellaneous activities	Surgery
Tuesday	Surgery	Visits or morning teaching session in Department	Half-day release course	Surgery
Wednesday	Surgery jointly with trainer	Visits and discussion	2-30-3.30 p.m. Teaching session	Surgery
Thursday	Surgery	Visits	Half-day	
Friday	Surgery	ANC with trainer	Visits 3-3.30 p.m. Teaching session	Surgery

Surgery appointments will be booked at a rate to be decided between the trainee and trainer. In the first six months of the GP year no pressure should be exerted on the trainee's appointment times at all. Visits will be arranged depending on appropriateness, follow-up situation, and practice demand.

Monday afternoon until evening surgery will be used for working on any arranged project or generally catching up on activities. The Wednesday morning surgery is a shared one in which either the trainee or trainer may do the consulting with the other sitting in.

Out-of-hours Duties

The philosophy behind this is that the trainee should do the same out-of-hours duties as his trainer. He will, therefore, have a half-day on a Thursday, but this may be changed from time to time if another partner is on holiday. He will do no surgeries or out-of-hours cover without a partner being available for advice and support if necessary.

The evening on duty extends from 6 p.m. to 8.30 a.m. and will normally be alternate Wednesdays with the trainer who will be covering the trainee on his duty night.

The weekend duty includes Friday evening, Saturday morning surgery and then on call until 8.30 a.m. on Monday. It will occur approximately twice in every three months, but will be specified, as different partners in turn will be covering this. At no time is the trainee actually built into the rota; he replaces one partner at a time in turn.

The trainee will also do an occasional Saturday morning surgery and visits when another practitioner is on duty for the weekend.

A separate list of duty dates is enclosed. If a date is inconvenient then there is no objection to the trainee arranging a 'swop' within the rota, provided that the trainer is agreeable.

In the university vacation when there is no half-day release, the trainee will normally do a surgery from 4-5 p.m.

He will also take late and emergency calls which arise after the end of morning surgery on Friday until after the evening surgery when the duty doctor for the weekend takes over.

As already mentioned, the above details are subject to variation in certain circumstances, particularly when one partner is on holiday. The main effect of this would be occasionally moving the half-day to a different day and having to do a night of duty rather than alternate Wednesdays.

APPENDIX L: PRACTICE CHECK LIST

The following check list is suggested as an *aide-mémoire* of questions to be asked when visiting a practice. If several practices are visited it may aid comparison if each question is scored 0-5, the highest total score showing the practice which is nearest your own ideal.

1. Partners

    (a) Age. Sex. Seniority.
    (b) Attitudes to each other.
    (c) Attitudes to wives (including yours).
    (d) Attitudes to the RCGP.
    (e) Special interests.
    (f) Research and/or publications.
    (g) Flexibility of approach.
    (h) Reason for partnership vacancy.

2. Premises

    (a) Health centre.
    (b) Privately owned—what is incoming partner's financial commitment?
    (c) Adequate space.
    (d) Own consulting-room.
    (e) Employed staff—receptionists, etc.
    (f) Employed practice nurse.
    (g) Attached staff (D/N, H/V, Social worker).
    (h) Equipment, e.g. ECG.
    (i) Furnishing and general impression.
    (j) Any special features.
    (k) Record system—quality of records.
    (l) Staff room.
    (m) Age-sex register.

3. Partnership Agreement

    (a) Is there one?
    (b) Time to parity.
    (c) Restrictive clauses.

4. Money

(a) Partnership accounts.
(b) Outside income, e.g. clinical assistantships.
(c) Is all income shared equally?
(d) Situation re seniority allowance, VT allowance, etc.
(e) Are employed staff paid realistic salaries?
(f) Is money being spent on improving the quality of care (e.g. pleasant premises, equipment, etc.)?

5. Workload

(a) Is work shared evenly?
(b) Is off-duty rota satisfactory?
(c) Is there an appointment system?
(d) Does the practice seem under pressure?
(e) Is there scope for expansion, e.g. clinical assistantship sessions, teaching, etc?
(f) Do the wives have to cover the telephone except when on call?

6. Holidays

(a) Amount per year.
(b) Study leave allowance.
(c) Restrictive clauses, e.g. only one partner away at a time.
(d) Sabbatical arrangements.

7. Housing

8. Schools

It must be emphasised that this list does not necessarily mean that items included are good or, if excluded, bad. It is purely an *aide-mémoire* and a help towards personal selection.

APPENDIX M: USEFUL ADDRESSES

Defence Bodies

1. The Medical Defence Union Ltd
   3 Devonshire Place, London W1N 2EA
   Tel. No. 01 486 6181

2. The Medical Protection Society Ltd
   50 Hallam Street, London W1N 6DE
   Tel. No. 01 637 0541

3. The Medical and Dental Defence Union of Scotland Ltd
   113 St Vincent Street
   Glasgow
   Tel. No. 041 221 8381

Associations and Colleges

4. Association of Police Surgeons of Great Britain
   17 East Park Parade
   Northampton NN1 4LE (Hon. Sec.)

5. British Medical Association
   General Medical Services Committee, including the Trainees' Sub-
     committee
   Personal Services Bureau
   Medical Practices Advisory Bureau
   BMA House, Tavistock Square
   London WC1H 9JP
   Tel. No. 01 387 4499

6. Medico-Legal Society
   71 Great Russell Street
   London WC1B 3BZ
   Tel. No. 01 405 0471

7. Medical Officers of Schools Association
   The Secretary, The Infirmary
   Christs Hospital, Horsham, Sussex RH13 7LT

8.   Medical Practitioners Union/ASTMD
       10-26A Jamestown Road, London NW1 7DI
       Tel. No. 01 267 4422

9.   Medical Women's Federation
       Tavistock House North, Tavistock Square
       London WC1H 9HX
       Tel. No. 01 387 7765

10.   Royal College of General Practitioners
       14 Princes Gate,
       London SW7 1PU
       Tel. No. 01 584 6262

11.   Society of Occupational Medicine
       c/o Royal College of Physicians
       11 St Andrew's Place, London NW1 4LE
       Tel. No. 01 486 2641

Government Departments

12.   Department of Health and Social Security
       Alexander Fleming House, Elephant & Castle
       London SE1 6BY
       Tel. No. 01 407 5522

13.   Northern Ireland: Department of Health and Social Services
       Dundonald House, Upper Newtownards Road, Belfast BT4 3SF
       Tel. No. 0232 650111

14.   Scottish Home and Health Department
       St Andrew's House, Edinburgh EH1 3DI
       Tel. No. 031 556 8501

15.   Welsh Office: Health and Social Work Department
       Pewil House, Greyfriars Road, Cardiff CF1 3RT
       Tel. No. 0222 44151

16.   HM Stationery Office
       PO Box 121
       Atlantic House, 45-50 Holborn Viaduct, London EC1
       Tel. No. 01 248 9876

GP Research and Postgraduate Activities

17.   British Postgraduate Medical Federation
(University of London)
14 Millman Mews, Millman Street, London WC1 3EJ
Tel. No. 01 405 2716

18.   Council for Postgraduate Medical Education, England and Wales
7 Marylebone Road, London NW1 5HA
Tel. No. 01 323 1289
   —N. Ireland: 5 Annadale Avenue, Belfast BT7 3JH
   Tel. No. 0232 646731
   —Scotland: 8 Queen Street, Edinburgh EH2 1JA
   Tel. No. 031 225 4365

19.   Medical Research Council
20 Park Crescent, London W1N 4AL
Tel. No. 01 636 5422

The Practice

20.   Association of Medical Secretaries
Tavistock House South, Tavistock Square,
London WC1H 9LN

21.   General Medical Council
44 Hallam Street, London W1N 6AE
Tel. No. 01 580 7642

22.   General Practice Finance Corporation
Tavistock House North, Tavistock Square,
London WC1 9JL
Tel. No. 01 387 5274

23.   Medical Practices Committee, England and Wales
Tavistock House South, Tavistock Square
London WC1
Tel. No. 01 387 8062
   —Scotland: St Andrew's House, Edinburgh EH1 3DI
   Tel. No. 031 556 8501